O1 Health Nursing

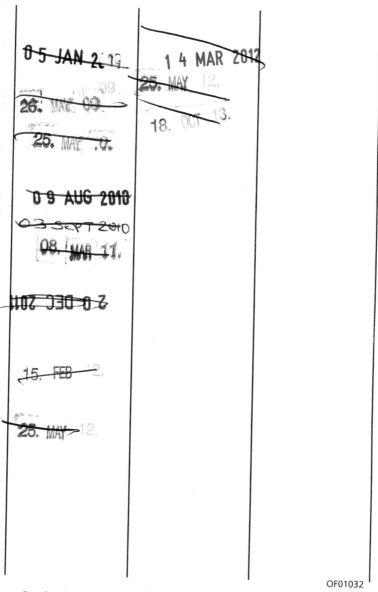

OF01032

Books should be returned to the SDH Library on or before
the date stamped above unless a renewal has been arranged

Salisbury District Hospital Library
Telephone: Salisbury (01722) 336262 extn. 4430 / 33
Out of hours answer machine in operation

Older People and Mental Health Nursing:
A Handbook of Care

Edited by

Rebecca Neno,
Barry Aveyard
and
Hazel Heath

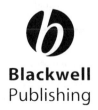

Blackwell
Publishing

Blackwell Publishing editorial offices:
Blackwell Publishing Ltd, 9600 Garsington Road, Oxford OX4 2DQ, UK
    Tel: +44 (0)1865 776868
Blackwell Publishing Inc., 350 Main Street, Malden, MA 02148-5020, USA
    Tel: +1 781 388 8250
Blackwell Publishing Asia Pty Ltd, 550 Swanston Street, Carlton, Victoria 3053, Australia
    Tel: +61 (0)3 8359 1011

First published 2007 by Blackwell Publishing Ltd

ISBN: 978-1-4051-5169-6

Library of Congress Cataloging-in-Publication Data

Older people and mental health nursing : a handbook of care / edited by Rebecca Neno, Barry
Aveyard, and Hazel Heath.
        p. ; cm.
    Includes bibliographical references and index.
ISBN: 978-1-4051-5169-6 (pbk. : alk. paper)
1. Psychiatric nursing. 2. Geriatric psychiatry. 3. Older people–Mental health. I. Neno, Rebecca.
II. Aveyard, Barry. III. Heath, Hazel B. M.
    [DNLM: 1. Mental Disorders—nursing. 2. Aged. 3. Geriatric Nursing—methods. 4. Psychiatric
Nursing—methods. WY 160 0435 2007]

    RC440.053 2007
    618.97'689—dc22

                                                                                    2007019846

A catalogue record for this title is available from the British Library

Set in 10/12.5 pt Palatino by Newgen Imaging Systems (P) Ltd, Chennai, India
Printed and bound in Singapore by Fabulous Printers Pte Ltd

For further information on Blackwell Publishing, visit our website:
www.blackwellnursing.com

Contents

Contributors

The Editors

Rebecca Neno MSc (Distinction), BSc(Hons), SPDN, Nprescriber, RN Dip HE, Cert Health Promotion, Primary Care Development Lead & Senior Lecturer in Primary Care, Thames Valley University London & Committee Member, RCN Mental Health and Older People's Forum

Barry Aveyard MA, BA(Hons), CertEd, RMN, RGN, RNT, Senior Lecturer, Faculty of Health and Wellbeing, Sheffield Hallam University, Sheffield & Committee Member, RCN Mental Health and Older People's Forum

Hazel Heath PhD, MSc Advanced Clinical Practice (Older People), BA(Hons), DipN(Lond), Cert Ed, FETC, RGN, RCNT, RNT, Independent Consultant on Nursing and Older People, Visiting Senior Fellow at City University, London and Consultant Editor Nursing to *The Journal of Dementia Care*

The Authors

Trevor Adams RMN, RGN, Cert Ed, CPN Cert, MSc, PhD, Pathway Leader, MSc Advanced Practice [Mental Health], European Institute of Health and Medical Sciences, University of Surrey, Guildford

Heide Baldwin RMN, ENB 941, 998, Locality Manager, Crawley and Horsham OPMH Services, Sussex Partnership and Chair of the RCN Mental Health and Older People's Forum

Gary Blatch RMN, MA, Dementia Nurse Specialist, South Essex Partnership Foundation Trust & Committee Member, RCN Mental Health and Older People's Forum

Elizabeth Collier BSc, MSc, RMN PGCE, Lecturer in Mental Health, School of Nursing, University of Salford, Manchester

Angela Cotter PhD, BSc (Soc Sci), Dip Health Ed, RN, Course Director, MPhil/ PhD Psychotherapy and Counselling, Regents College, London

Sue Davies PhD, MSc, BSc, RGN, RHV, Honorary Reader, University of Sheffield

Jan Dewing RGN, MN, BSc, RNT, Dip Nurs Ed, Dip Nurs, Independent Consultant Nurse; also Associate Fellow Practice Development, RCN Institute, Associate

Lecturer, School of Education, University of Ulster, and Visiting Fellow, School of Health, Community & Education Studies, University of Northumbria

Peter Draper RGN, PhD, Dip Theol Min, Senior Lecturer in Nursing, Department of Applied Health Studies, Faculty of Health and Social Care, The University of Hull

Christine Eberhardie TD, MSc, RN, RNT, ILTM, MIHM, Honorary Principal Lecturer, Faculty of Health and Social Sciences, St George's, University of London

Denise Forte Dip Applied Sciences (Nursing), MSc Gerontology, PGCEA, RGN, RSCN, Principal Lecturer, Gerontology, Faculty of Health and Social Care Sciences, Kingston University & St George's, University of London

Steve Iliffe FRCGP, Reader in General Practice, Department of Primary Care & Population Sciences, University College London

Jill Manthorpe MA, FRSA, Professor of Social Work, Co-Director of the Social Care Workforce Research Unit, King's College London

Sarah McGeorge RGN, RMN, DipN, BSc(Hons), PGDip, Nurse Consultant, Mental Health Services for Older People, Tees, Esk and Wear Valleys NHS Trust, Honorary Lecturer and Doctoral Student, University of Teesside

Wilfred McSherry RGN, PhD, Senior Lecturer in Nursing, Faculty of Health and Social Care, The University of Hull

Henry Minardi MSc, BSc, DipN, DipCounselling&Supervision, CertEd, RGN, RMN, Consultant Nurse, Liaison Psychiatry for Older Adults, Central and North West London Mental Health NHS Trust, London

Tina Naldrett MSc, RGN, RMN, Deputy Clinical Lead, Devon Primary Care Trust

Lynne Phair MA, BSc(Hons) Nursing, RMN, RGN, DPNS, prescriber Consultant Nurse, Older People, West Sussex Primary Care Trust, Fellow University of Brighton, Fellow Institute of Leadership and Management

Tony Ryan PhD, Senior Lecturer, Faculty of Health & Wellbeing, Sheffield Hallam University

Irene Schofield MSc (Gerontology), RGN, RNT, Research Fellow, School of Nursing, Midwifery and Community Health, Glasgow Caledonian University

Michael Tullett RGN, RMN, MSc (Gerontology), Senior Lecturer, Thames Valley University, Faculty of Health & Human Sciences, Slough, Berkshire

Roger Watson PhD, RN, FIBiol, FRSA, Professor of Nursing, School of Nursing and Midwifery, The University of Sheffield

Diane Wells MPhil, RGN, BA, Dip Soc Stud, Dip Soc Res, Dip Nurs, RNT, Cassel Certificate in Psychosocial Nursing, Senior Lecturer

Foreword

This is an important text in bringing together the complex and diverse challenges for nurses working with older people with mental health needs. Across adult care, in acute hospitals, communities and care homes, older people will present with either pre-existing health conditions or demonstrate signs of deterioration of mental well-being.

Nursing in 21st-century health care requires practitioners to have a wide and comprehensive knowledge of a breadth of issues which both enable them to deliver better care. This will be achieved through effective assessment, complex care management and ensuring that fundamental care principles such as nutrition are received. Also, nurses will need to have an understanding of the legislative, and socio-political, cultural, sexual and end-of-life issues which are important underpinning themes of nursing today.

Nurses are key in delivering care and promoting well-being for older people with mental health needs. It is therefore essential that they develop the clinical skills and competencies to deliver effective care. In addition, as clinical leaders, nurses can be effective role models by demonstrating positive attitudes to promote well-being and management of mental illness.

This text brings together a range of nursing and other experts who have articulated the essence of knowledge and clinical competence which will equip readers with the requisite skills and knowledge to be the best and give the best.

Globally, contemporary health care is changing at a rapid pace, and this book will enable nurses, as the largest component of the workforce, to prepare, understand and rise to the challenge of working in partnership across the health- and social-care spectrum to make a real difference to older people and their families.

Deborah Sturdy, RN, MSc (Econ)
Nurse Advisor for Older People
Department of Health
London

Introduction

Mental health in later life is influenced by a complex set of biological, psychological and social interactions. As such, nurses need to be aware of how each of these influences may affect the older person with mental health needs. In addition to these influences, older people may also have to cope with societal assumptions that ageing automatically brings mental decline, and that no treatments are available. Nurses need to be able to challenge such views and assumptions, and to do this they must have adequate knowledge relating to the natural ageing process and skills in communication to be able to get their message across. These are seen as fundamental principles of mental health care for older adults and, of course, will be explored further within this book.

The underpinning concepts and approaches in this book value individual persons within the context of their lives, experiences and relationships. Mental health is seen as an integral aspect of overall health and as a continuum between wellness and illness. Traditional views of mental ill-health as disease can lead to people who experience this being labelled as 'different', with all the stigma this can attract. Rather, as Crump (1998, pp. 172–173) argues, we acknowledge that

'we all have both wellness and illness . . . mental health and mental distress are a continuum on which we all move back and forth, attempting to strike the right balance . . . People who have moved along the continuum away from health are still the same people but are now distressed and in need of support and understanding. The difference is not merely political correctness: it is crucial to how we perceive mental health nursing and, more importantly how we perceive those who find themselves requiring mental health support.'

This book focuses on the knowledge and key skills which practitioners require or must have, to work effectively with older people who have, or are at risk of developing, mental health needs. The text is aimed primarily at nurses working in all settings and all types of roles, but, acknowledging the intrinsically interdisciplinary nature of older people's services, much of the content is relevant to all disciplines. The content relevant to older people's mental health and care is broadly applicable, and the social policy, legislation and details of specific services are relevant to the UK.

It is intended that this book will enable practitioners to develop their knowledge and skills through the completion of the practice examples found within most chapters. These examples are meant to be thought-provoking, allowing readers to link theoretical concepts with their practice and ultimately improve the delivery of care.

The book is divided into five sections, to assist the reader in navigating the text.

Part 1 sets the context for the book; it explores the background, historical perspectives and influences of mental health care in later life. This section is designed to provide the foundation of the book; understanding the history and origins of elements of care and practice should assist practitioners in the mission of moving forward and developing practice further.

Part 2 focuses on helping older individuals, and includes chapters relating to:

- older individuals and mental health;
- normal age changes that influence mental health;
- values underpinning support and care;
- legal and ethical frameworks within which mental health care takes place;
- the practical implications of the legal and ethical frameworks by exploring some dilemmas in mental health nursing;
- assessing older people with mental health needs, including the importance of developing therapeutic relationships.

Part 3 focuses on some aspects which have traditionally been neglected in mental health care, including:

- culture, religion and spirituality;
- intimacy, sex and sexuality;
- nutrition;
- palliative and end-of-life care.

Part 4 details specific mental health issues for older people; these include:

- acute mental health issues;
- delirium;
- enduring mental health issues;
- depression in later life;
- dementia.

The final section explores future trends in older people's mental health and offers ideas as to how nursing may develop, and is developing, to address these.

The contributing authors of this book have considerable expertise in the care of older people and/or mental health care. We would like to extend our thanks to all authors who have contributed to this book and have worked hard to ensure their chapters are robust and contemporary. As such, we hope that this book will ultimately make a contribution to enhanced care and support for older people with mental health needs.

Rebecca Neno, Hazel Heath, Barry Aveyard

Reference

Crump, A. (1998) Disease or distress. In: *Caring for Older People: Developing Specialist Practice* (J. Marr and B. Kershaw, eds). London, Arnold, pp. 165–189.

Part 1
CONTEXT

Chapter 1
Background and Influences

Rebecca Neno, Barry Aveyard, Hazel Heath and Heide Baldwin

Introduction

There is one thing in life that is inevitable – ageing; and with ageing come biological, psychological and sociological changes and adjustments. As advances in knowledge, technology and health care continue, both life expectancy and lifespan are increasing. Lifespan is the maximum time a person can live, currently 122 years, whereas life expectancy is the average time a person can expect to live, currently 76 years for males and 81 years for females, within the UK (Official National Statistics, 2006). The increase in both lifespan and life expectancy has brought about considerable demographic changes for developed countries such as the UK. By 2030, the UK will have seen radical changes in its population structure. It has been predicted that the number of people over the age of 85 will double, resulting in a disproportionate cohort of old old age. Consequently, the average life expectancy is now nearing maximum lifespan.

As a result, health and social policy has heightened the awareness of public health and government initiatives often focus on the promotion of health and well-being. In England, the National Service Framework for Older People (Department of Health, 2001) has a standard dedicated to health and exercise in later life (standard 8). The Welsh Strategy for Older People (Welsh Assembly Government, 2003) aims to develop an evidence-based action programme of health promotion for older people and through community health and well-being planning, ensure local government takes a strategic approach to older people issues and responds to an ageing society. In 2006, the Scottish Executive consulted on a strategy for an ageing population; once again the consultation included the maintenance of health and well-being in later life (Scottish Executive, 2006). Similarly, policies within Northern Ireland also focus upon the promotion of health and activity in later life (Older People Improving Health, 2006). This change in policy focus is reflective of the move away from a curative approach of ill-health, to one of wellbeing and the management of long-term illness conditions.

Traditionally, most health and wellness strategies have been aimed at physical health, and in comparison few have focused on mental health and well-being. While it is important to stress that most older people, as at any age, do not develop a mental health need, their mental health and well-being should be given equal emphasis to physical health needs. This will become increasingly important in the future as the numbers of older people increase. Age Concern and the Mental Health Foundation (2006) claim that, unless mental health and well-being in later life are promoted, as many as three million older people may develop mental health needs by 2031.

Psychological perspectives on mental health

Despite ageing being inevitable, the development of mental health needs at any stage in the lifespan is not. However, myths remain that as a person ages, cognitive changes occur which negatively affect intelligence, creativity and memory. While it cannot be argued that some changes take place within the brain as a person ages (see Chapter 3), it is wrong to assume that all older people will become forgetful and develop a dementia-related condition. Although there is some agreement on the biological changes occurring in ageing, there is little research-based agreement on the psychological dimensions (Daly, 1999), despite numerous research attempts. The difficulty with research studies is that, while attempting to provide a generalisable snapshot of the reality of mental health in later life, they cannot always reflect or provide answers to meeting individual needs (Daly, 1999). Adopting a person-centred and biographical approach to care can be crucial to planning services and meeting individual care needs. The major areas of psychological investigation and research include the decline of learning abilities, memory, personality changes and intelligence. All are considered to impact upon abilities in later life (see Chapter 3).

The first distinct contribution of psychology to the study of ageing is credited to Sir Francis Galton (1822–1911) who, among his other works, launched the first large-scale collection of empirical data across the lifespan. At this time, research into intelligence quotients (IQ) compared younger people with older people in laboratory conditions, and unsurprisingly these studies demonstrated a significant decline in ability in later life. This theory proposed that from birth, the individual learns and grows until adulthood, after which there is a long stage of consolidation, followed by a stage of decline, culminating in death. We now know that laboratory tests involving quick responses actually test motor function, rather than IQ, and such work has declined in importance since the emergence of developmental psychology.

Jung (1875–1961) was one of the first psychologists to define later life as having a purpose of its own. He described the first half of life as orientated to biological and social issues and the second half of life characterised by inner discovery. Jung identified this as a developmental process by which the person becomes more unique and better able to use inner resources to pursue personal aims. Overall, within current gerontological theory, it is accepted that, as a person ages, personality does not change. Similarly, changes to both short-term and long-term memory are thought to occur with the natural ageing process (see Chapter 3), but it is thought that these changes do not necessarily impact upon the person's life, and often those complaining of poor memory in later life also report poor memory ability in earlier years.

Older people's mental health

There exists a broad assumption that older people's mental health is all about dementia. This is untrue. According to Age Concern and the Mental Health Foundation (2006), depression is the most common mental health condition in later life, and there are currently 2.4 million older people in the UK with depression severe enough to impair their quality of life (see Chapter 16). Aside from depression, older people are also prone to other mental health conditions: 5% of the population aged over 65 have dementia (Department of Health, 2001); 20% of older adults in an acute hospital environment will develop delirium (British Geriatrics Society, 2005) (see Chapter 14), and 1% of the older population within the UK have schizophrenia (Rodriguez-Ferra and Vassilas, 1998) (see Chapter 15).

While wishing to avoid 'labelling' or to focus merely on diagnosis, it is important to recognise that older people experience a broad range of mental health issues, and these may also include:

- dementia of varying types (Chapter 17);
- schizophrenia and paranoid states (Chapter 15);
- bipolar disorders (Chapter 15);
- anxiety states;
- stress-related disorders, post-traumatic stress;
- the effects of alcohol or drug misuse.

Apart from dementia, many areas of older people's mental health have been particularly neglected, and this may be attributed to prejudicial perceptions of old age. Dyson (2006) claims that alcohol misuse among older people is a neglected issue within mental health care. While it could be argued that the incidence of alcohol misuse is underestimated in all age groups, older people are notably absent in policy priorities (Galpin, 2004). For example, the Alcohol Harm Reduction Strategy for England (Strategy Unit, 2004) focuses on young binge drinkers and alcohol-dependent people of working age. Mental health and alcohol misuse are closely related and can interact through a cycle whereby stressors or mental health needs can increase alcohol consumption which, in turn, can affect mental health. Mixing alcohol with some prescribed drugs can be particularly dangerous for older people. Specialist services are limited, and the number of older people accessing these is low (Alcohol Concern, 2002 calculate that only 7% of specialist alcohol service users are over 60 years of age), but older people who do access treatment are able to alter their drinking patterns (Ward, 2003).

Another neglected area includes post-traumatic stress disorder (PTSD), labelled as 'shell shock', 'battle fatigue' or even 'weak willed', which was common during and after the two World Wars. It was first identified by the psychiatrist WH Rivers working at Craiglockhart hospital in Edinburgh during the First World War. Working with soldiers suffering from psychological trauma, he developed the phrase war neurosis (Rivers, 1918). However, it was not until the latter part of the 20th century when research documented the extreme psychological reactions to major disasters that the underlying psychological processes developed. Now conceptualised as a catastrophic stressor outside the range of usual human experience (Farnsworth, 2002), PTSD is now more widely recognised among older people, and a range of psychotherapeutic and pharmacological treatments are available (Mason, 2005). There is perhaps a view in society that ideas around stress and psychological trauma are alien to older people, and that the 'older generation' just 'get on with it'. However, this is a likely stereotype with no real supporting evidence.

There are also groups of older people whose mental health needs are commonly under-recognised. These include older people who are homeless and those in prison. These are discussed further in Chapter 18.

The development of mental health services for older people

The history of mental health care is long and complex, but it is important to understand the legacy that current services have inherited as some influences from this remain today. Some of the earliest documentation refers to the founding of the Bethlehem Hospital in London in 1327 for the mentally distracted (McMillan, 1996). One of the first attempts to legislate in the field of mental health care was the 1774 Madhouses Act; this act introduced the concept of inspection of madhouses by commissioners (Wright, 1999).

The development of the lunatic asylum can be attributed to the 1845 Lunacy Act. This legislation led to the compulsory founding of asylums in every county borough in the UK. While with hindsight we tend to see the old asylums as very unpleasant places, in 1845 the idea of care for 'lunatics' was seen as very progressive and innovative. In 1957, the Percy Report claimed that there needed to be a much more therapeutic approach to mental health and monitoring of asylums. This report led to the 1959 Mental Health Act, which is often regarded as setting the foundations for modern mental health care (Nolan, 1992).

The development of neuroleptic drugs in the 1950s also played a revolutionary role in the development of mental health care. While there are without doubt many issues around the use of neuroleptic drugs, and clear evidence exists that they have at times been misused, there remains little doubt that they did revolutionise care. They brought about the demise of regular use of straitjackets and locked wards in 'mental hospitals'. They also slowly led to the development of community mental health care. It took nearly 50 years for the old psychiatric hospitals to close their doors, but it is now unlikely that people entering mental health care now will spend the rest of their lives in institutional settings.

Kitwood (1997) highlighted that the historical approach to older people in institutions was to 'warehouse' them (and this is discussed further in

Chapter 17). The suggestion was that they were cared for in places of safety where their basic human needs were provided for, but little else. Even today, institutional care can persist in any environment where staff do not focus upon the needs of the individual or do not question rituals. As the move towards community care developed in the 1970s, community services developed in an unstructured and disorganised way, and health and social services saw the needs of those with mental health conditions very differently (Phair, 1999). Despite the fact that there were some areas of excellent development, there were nonetheless a number of tragedies involving those with mental health needs, the most well known being the death of Jonathan Zito, who was murdered by Christopher Clunis on an underground station for no apparent reason. The enquiry into Jonathan Zito's death concluded that poor communication between health and social services and a lack of effective care coordination were contributing factors. As a result, an emphasis upon joint local services for people with mental health needs became a government priority, and thus the Care Programme Approach came to fruition. The Care Programme Approach should ensure that all older people with mental health needs, living in the community:

- have a key worker;
- have regular reviews of the care package undertaken by the multiagency team;
- have all care assessed and that care is reviewed in a systematic way.

A further requirement of the Care Programme Approach was to make the person's perspective central to any plan of treatment or care. This has been affirmed as a central component in the Review of the Care Programme Approach 2006 (Department of Health, 2006). The notion of person-centred care has become well established within both health and social care professional frameworks and is an idea associated with the groundbreaking work of Tom Kitwood (1997). Person-centred care aims to break the traditional approach to care, which often involved ritualised approaches. It aims to ensure that each person is cared for in an individualised manner. It is a concept that is now well established in care provision and underpins many government documents produced by the four countries of the UK (Department of Health, 2001; Welsh National Assembly, 2003).

At the start of the millennium, there was a shift in the focus of person-centred care. The Institute for Health Care Improvement (2001) broadened the remit to 'care that is truly person-centred considers the persons cultural traditions, their preferences and values and their family situation and lifestyle'. This shift has been accepted as progression, involving a radical movement from a highly individualised therapeutic approach to a social and political strategy.

It would be hard to disagree that person-centred care is an important way of looking to develop standards of care for older people. The challenge is to actually ensure that it is a reality and not rhetoric. Some researchers (Aveyard and Davies, 2006; Nolan et al., 2006) among others have begun to explore the notion of Relationship-Centred Care; this approach suggests that to achieve person-centred care for older people, there needs to be a consideration of the needs of relatives and care staff as well as those of the person themselves. It is suggested that if there is a sense of well-being for all involved in care, then the outcome for the person being cared for will be much more person-centred in nature. The rationale for this change is based on increased recognition of the need to develop a systematic approach towards care (Adams, 2005). The foundation for change is that interaction in health and social care frequently requires the involvement of three or more people. It is less common to be dealing with only one individual in care. Where this triangle of care exists, various authors have commented on the risk of alienating the least able person where the focus is upon just one person (Biggs, 1993; Twigg and Atkin, 1994; Adams, 2005).

Relationship-centred care needs to consider the whole picture. There are risks associated with this, specifically where the person receiving care is unable to communicate their wishes and needs. The risk of losing the person in the development of relationship-centered care is recognised by Nolan et al. (2003, 2004). He is explicit in identifying that the inner subjectivity of the individual remains core, but in addition to these, others must be considered. Nolan et al. (2003) argues that there are prerequisites for good relationships, and he terms them as the 'senses framework'. The six senses are security, continuity, belonging, purpose, fulfillment and significance. The need for security includes feeling safe in both the receiving of and delivery of competent and sensitive care. The sense of continuity is both that of personhood, of having a history in life with positive past experiences that are recognised and valued. The sense of belonging is reciprocal, with opportunities to form meaningful relationships or feel part of a team, whereas a sense of purpose is found in the agreement of clear goals that are inspirational to the practitioner, the client and their carer or family. The achievement of meaningful and valued goals brings satisfaction or the sense of fulfillment, without which the relationship is empty; and in recognising the person, be that client, carer or professional, there is a feeling of significance in the role (Adams, 2005).

The contribution of nursing

Effective health care for older people requires the input of specialist professionals from a range of disciplines including medicine, physiotherapy, occupational therapy, speech and language therapy, nutrition, pharmacy, podiatry, as well as nurses who make their own distinct contribution.

Heath's (2006a) research highlights that good nurses bring to their work, among other inputs, an understanding of:

- health and disease processes – physical, emotional, social, spiritual – and how these interact;
- a broad range of treatment options including the effects and side-effects of medicines and also a variety of therapeutic interventions.

Good nurses:

- focus on supporting individuals as they experience changes in health or functioning;
- develop an understanding of individuals through person-centred and biographical approaches;
- learn about individuals, their health and their life situations through skilled assessment (see Chapter 8);
- are able to help others through building and developing therapeutic relationships (see Chapter 8)

The work of good nurses encompasses:

- creating and maintaining environments of care;
- dealing with emergencies or accidents;
- risk assessment and management;
- rehabilitation/re-enablement;
- preventative and anticipatory care;
- health promotion;
- end-of-life care, symptom relief, family support;
- therapeutics (e.g. reminiscence);
- advocacy;
- and a range of skills they develop as a result of their professional training and experience such as ethical decision-making and not panicking in emergencies.

Fundamentally, Heath's research concludes that 'the presence of an astute, skilled, knowledgeable and experienced Registered Nurse offers a perceptual awareness that can "read situations", identify problems and interpret these in terms of the potential consequences and actions needed' (Heath 2006b, p. 21).

Assessment is and has to be a foundation of excellence in nursing care of older adults, and particularly those with mental health needs (see Chapter 8). A thorough and robust assessment is determined by the possession and employment of excellent and therapeutic communication skills. This is frequently where nurses have difficulty, citing lack of time, often, as a barrier to communication. Such barriers disempower both the nurse and client when decisions need to be made. These decisions are even more complex if the client lacks capacity (see Chapter 6) and consensus surrounding issues of consent is incredibly difficult to achieve. Competence in communication and the ability to undertake a robust and comprehensive assessment including those areas which nurses often find difficult to discuss, such as cultural influences or spirituality (Chapter 9), intimacy, sex or sexuality (Chapter 10) and death and dying (Chapter 12) are fundamental skills in working with older people who have mental health issues. It remains a challenge for nurses to ensure that older people with mental-health needs and those who may lack capacity are not excluded from decision-making and participation in activities.

A current challenge for nursing must be to provide therapeutic, stimulating care that looks to maintaining psychological as well as physical well-being, regardless of the care setting the older person is in. Particularly in communal care settings, this entails consciously rejecting approaches influenced by historical values of containment and conformity. As dementia care has become more community-orientated, and with an increasing number of purpose-built dementia care units within the public, private and charity sector, attention has increasingly turned to architecture and design as a way of contributing to development in quality of dementia care, (Cantley and Wilson, 2002). The Foundation for Assistive Technology (2005) has researched how technology might be incorporated into design for dementia care to develop independence for people with dementia and has suggested that controlling elements such as light levels and background noise allow residents in care homes to experience a higher level of well-being. Chalfont (2006) has taken design out of the built environment and considered the use of therapeutic outdoor environments. His work suggests that garden environments are powerful ways of allowing people with dementia to connect with nature and that this can increase their ability to sense feel, and communicate in a meaningful way. It is of course inevitable that good design and planning will cost money, and ways will need to be sought to ensure adequate funding if good design is a principle that will be taken forward. There appears to be increasing literature about the impact of environment on dementia care, and, while principles of good design in dementia care may be transferable, the lack of research on the impact of environments on people with enduring mental health conditions would appear to reflect the lack of literature around aspects of older people's mental health generally.

There is also an increasing interest in a variety of therapeutic approaches and interventions, for example on therapy in therapeutic work for people living with dementia (Feil, 2002) The philosophy of validation therapy is to 'validate' or accept the values, beliefs and 'reality' of the person with dementia, even if what they are saying appears confused or disorientated. Validation allows the carer to let the person with dementia express their feelings and emotions, without challenging them even if what they are expressing is clearly muddled. While not encouraging the carer to lie to the person, it does allow them to be supportive without having to challenge the reality of the person. An example of this might be a person with dementia who regularly talks about a parent as if they are living, although they may have been dead for some time. The carer could challenge this and share the reality of the situation, or they could decide that this may well be distressing and therefore decide to allow the person to continue with the conversation accepting that it is their reality.

Other therapies now widely accepted include pet therapy and drama therapy. The introduction of pets into long-stay care facilities has been proven to decrease stress, improve health and well-being and increase social interaction between residents (Richeson, 2003; Cangelosi and Embrey, 2006). Recent research has also demonstrated that pet therapy can help people with schizophrenia feel more motivated and improve their quality of life (Nathans-Barel et al., 2005). For those with Alzheimer's disease, drama therapy has also been found to be useful. Garrett (2006) highlights the aim of drama therapy to stimulate the senses, muscles and nerves, to spark a sensory memory and to ignite imagination. Drama activities are, first of all, concrete and sensory. They include improvisation, theatre games, storytelling and enactment and always a movement component. Only those trained in such activities should undertake them, but nurses should be aware of their potential in the overall management of older people with mental health needs.

There is great potential for nurses to address and resolve issues of older people's mental health. All nurses will be aware that working with older people with mental health issues can be not only incredibly challenging but also incredibly rewarding. To move both care and services forward, nurses must have a thorough understanding of the influences on our work, whether they be historical or current. Having harnessed this understanding, we must now move forward to ensure that all older people with mental health issues, in all their diversity, receive timely and evidence-based care that is the very best we can offer.

References

Adams, T. (2005) From person centred care to relationship centred care. *Generations Review* **15** (1), 4–7.

Age Concern and Mental Health Foundation (2006) *Promoting Mental Health and Well-Being in Later Life*. London, Age Concern and Mental Health Foundation.

Alcohol Concern (2002) *Report on the Mapping of Alcohol Services in England*. London, Alcohol Concern.

Aveyard, B. and Davies, S. (2006) Moving forward together: evaluation of an action group involving staff and relatives within a nursing home for older people with dementia. *International Journal of Nursing Older People* **1** (2), 95–104.

Biggs, S. (1993) User participation and interprofessional collaboration in community care. *Interprofessional Care* **7** (2), 151–160.

British Geriatrics Society (2005) *Guidelines for the prevention, diagnosis and management of delirium in older people in hospital*. London, British Geriatrics Society. http://www.bgs.org.uk/publications/publication%20Downloads/Delirium-2006.Doc

Cangelosi, P. and Embrey, C. (2006) The healing power of dogs: Cocoa's story. *Journal of Psychosocial Nursing and Mental Health Services* **44** (1), 17–20.

Cantley, C. and Wilson, R. (2002) *Put Yourself in my Place: Designing and Managing Care Homes for People with Dementia*. Bristol, UK, Policy Press.

Chalfont Garuth (2006) *Therapeutic nature designs*. http://www.chalfontdesign.com

Daly, S. (1999) Exploring the myths and stereotypes of mental health in old age. In: *Older People, Nursing and Mental Health* (Darby, S., Marr, J., Crump, A. and Scurfield, M., eds). Oxford, Butterworth-Heinemann.

Department of Health (2001) *National Service Framework for Older People*. London, Department of Health.

Department of Health (2006) *Reviewing the Care Programme Approach*. London, Department of Health.

Dyson, J. (2006) Alcohol misuse and older people. *Nursing Older People* **18** (7), 32–35.

Farnsworth, K. (2002) *The Hidden Injury: Post Traumatic Stress Disorder in Dementia*. Rhonda, The Farnsworth Consultancies.

Feil, N. (2002) *The Validation Breakthrough: Simple Techniques for Communicating with People with Alzheimer's Type Dementia*. Sydney, MacLennan & Petty.

Foundation for Assistive Technology (2005) Assitive technology in dementia care. http://www.fastuk.org/home.php

Galpin, D. (2004) Older people drink too. *Community Care*, 9–15 December, 40–41.

Garrett, K. (2006) *Drama therapy can coax Alzheimer's patients back to reality, briefly*. http://www.mediarelations.k-state.edu/WEB/News/Webzine/aging/dramatherapy.html

Heath, H. (2006a) *The work of registered nurses and care assistants with older people in nursing homes: can the outcomes be distinguished?* Ph.D. thesis, Brunel University, London.

Heath, H. (2006b) No substitute for Nurses. *Nursing Standard* **21** (10), 18–21.

Institute of Health Care Improvement (2001) *Crossing the Quality Chasm: A New Health System for the 21st Century*. London, Institute of Health Care Improvement.

Kitwood, T. (1997) *Dementia Reconsidered*. Buckingham, UK, Open University Press.

McMillan, I. (1996) Years of bedlam. *Nursing Times* **92** (47), 62–63.

Mason, A. (2005) Recurrence of post traumatic stress disorder. *Nursing Older People* **17** (6), 24–29.

Nathans-Barel, I., Feldman, P., Berger, B., Modai, I. and Silver, H. (2005) Animal-assisted therapy ameliorates anhedonia in schizophrenia patients: a controlled pilot study. *Psychotherapy and Psychosomatics* **74** (1), 31–35.

Nolan, M., Davies, S. and Brown, J. (2006) Transitions in care homes: towards relationship-centred care using the 'senses framework'. *Quality in Ageing* **7** (3), 5–12.

Nolan, M., Davies, S., Brown, J., Keady, J. and Nolan, J. (2004) Beyond person centred care a new vision for gerontological nursing. *Journal of Clinical Nursing* **13** (s1), 45–53.

Nolan, M., Lundh, U., Grant, G. and Keady, J. (2003) *Partnerships in Family Care*. Buckingham, UK, Open University Press.

Nolan, P. (1992) *A History of Mental Health Nursing*. London, Chapman & Hall.

Official National Statistics (2006) *Life expectancy*. http://www.statistics.gov.uk/cci/nugget.asp?id=168

Older People Improving Health (2006) *Improving health of older people*. http://www.publichealthmatters.org/olderpeople.htm

Phair, L. (1999) Mental health. In: *Healthy Ageing Nursing Older People* (Heath, H. and Schofield, I., eds). London, Mosby, pp. 407–433.

Richeson, N. (2003) Effects of animal-assisted therapy on agitated behaviors and social interactions of older adults with dementia. *American Journal of Alzheimer's Disease and Other Dementias* **18** (6), 353–358.

Rivers, W.H. (1918) On the repression of the war experience. *The Lancet* 2 February, **1**, 172–177.

Rodriguez-Ferra, S. and Vassilas, C. (1998) Older people with schizophrenia: providing services for neglected groups. *British Medical Journal* **317**, 293–294.

Scottish Executive (2006) *Strategy for an ageing population*. http://www.scotland.gov.uk/News/Releases/2006/03/13102201

Strategy Unit (2004) *Alcohol Harm Reduction Strategy for England*. London, Cabinet Office.

Twigg, J. and Atkin, K. (1994) *Carers Perceived: Policy and Practice*. Buckingham, UK, Open University Press.

Ward, M. (2003) *Caring for Someone with an Alcohol Problem*. Revised Edition. London, Age Concern.

Welsh Assembly Government (2006) *National Service Framework for Older People in Wales*. Welsh Assembly Government, Cardiff.

Wright, D. (1999) *The history of mental health nursing*. http://www.shef.ac.uk/~nmhuk/mhnurs/mhnhome.html

Part 2
HELPING OLDER INDIVIDUALS

Chapter 2
Older Individuals and Mental Health

Sue Davies and Tony Ryan

Introduction

Working effectively with older people with mental health conditions requires an understanding of the experience of old age. Within this chapter, we will be drawing on research evidence to provide an overview of common experiences in later life. We begin with a brief consideration of the main conditions that result in mental illness among older people, with a particular focus on dementia and depression. This is followed by an overview of the main factors that shape experiences of ageing and influence mental health and well-being during this life stage. We then consider some of the many changes that older people experience in their lives and health and look at the experiences of family members when an older person has mental health needs. Finally, we provide a summary of some of the services available to support older people with mental health conditions and their carers.

The mental health of older people

As in any time of life, older people can experience a range of mental health conditions and difficulties, both organic (where there is identifiable brain malfunction) and functional (mental illnesses not due to structural abnormalities of the brain). These include dementia, depression and adjustment reactions, schizophrenia, substance misuse, delirium and anxiety disorders (Ferguson and Keady, 2001). There are, however, specific aetiologies which predispose older people to particular forms of mental health conditions. Dementia is the name given to the signs or symptoms associated with a range of primary brain disorders or neurological impairments. These disorders are numerous. Typically dementia can be caused by Alzheimer's disease, vascular disease, stroke or HIV/AIDS. The signs and symptoms of dementia are likely to include memory loss and confusion, or behavioural and personality change. These symptoms are progressive and can be severe. The prevalence of dementia rises steadily with age, with one-quarter of those aged 85 or over being diagnosed. It is estimated that over one-third of people with dementia continue to live at home with their families (Melzer et al., 1997). However, mental health conditions for older people are not confined to the so-called 'organic' diseases. Anxiety and, more significantly, depression are also features of daily life for many older people. Although major depression appears to decline with age, studies suggest that between one in ten and one in six older people indicate signs of major depression (Godfrey and Denby, 2004).

One of the major difficulties facing health-care staff working with older people is that many of the signs and symptoms of different mental health conditions are similar. For instance, while older people suffering from anxiety may show signs of fearfulness, distress and panic, these symptoms are also consistent with depression. However, older people who are depressed may also show signs of lack of appetite, poor self-worth, low self-esteem and low motivation. Older people with depressive illness or anxiety may also show signs of memory loss and confusion, which can of course be confused with one of the dementias (Manthorpe and Iliffe, 2006). Other disorders, such as delirium and cognitive decline, can also be confused with the above (Insel and Badger, 2002). These prevailing notions of older people's mental health are, however, problematic. While it can be recognised that organic and functional decline provides us with the primary reason for symptom or behavioural changes which a person may display, the sources of mental health conditions for older people are also firmly rooted in the social and psychological environment. Furthermore, the experience of dementia, depression and anxiety, their trajectory and life impact is shaped by a number of factors diffuse in scope. Within this chapter it is our intention to locate the experience of older people with mental health conditions within a wider social and psycho-social framework. With this in mind, we will now consider experiences of growing older and the range of factors likely to impact on mental well-being during this life phase.

Experiences of ageing and mental illness

Ageing is a very individual experience, although there are a number of common themes in accounts of growing older. For example, old age is often encountered as a time of multiple losses, requiring adaptation to new situations and circumstances. Similarly, individual experiences of mental illness in later life are also unique: nonetheless, there will be some experiences that are common to many people with particular mental health needs. An understanding of both the range and commonalities of these experiences are essential in order to support older people and their families effectively.

The process of ageing involves a combination of biological, psychological and social changes. Many of these changes are quite challenging and can be compounded by the presence of a mental health condition, creating what has been termed 'double jeopardy' (Age Concern, 2006). However, mental health conditions are not a normal and inevitable part of the ageing process. The majority of older people enjoy good mental health and continue to make a valuable contribution to society.

Evidence about the factors that affect mental health and well-being has increased in recent years. We now know much more, for example, about the link between social isolation and mental illness. In 2006, the charity Age Concern, in partnership with the Mental Health Foundation, published the first report of the UK enquiry into mental health and well-being in later life (Age Concern, 2006). This report draws on a comprehensive review of policy and literature and identifies ways to promote mental health in old age. The enquiry also invited nearly 900 older people and carers to share their views and experiences of what helps to promote well-being in later life, together with more than 150 professionals and organisations. The review identified five main areas that influence mental health for older people:

- discrimination;
- participation in meaningful activity;
- relationships;
- physical health;
- poverty.

Each of these will be discussed in more detail to highlight some of the positive steps that nurses can take to enable older people to maintain good mental health.

Discrimination

Ageist attitudes, whereby older people are perceived as somehow inferior to other adults, are widespread in the UK and have a strong influence on the extent to which older people are able to enjoy full participation in society. These attitudes are based on the false belief that older age is inevitably a time of physical and mental decline. On the contrary, as we have already suggested, many older people live varied and fulfilling lives, valuing their independence and continuing to make an important contribution. In a report entitled 'How ageist is Britain?', the charity Age Concern provides evidence that ageism is the most prevalent form of discrimination in Great Britain (Age Concern, 2005). A nationally representative survey which provided the basis for the report found that 29% of respondents had experienced age discrimination, and those aged 55 and over were twice as likely to have experienced ageism compared with any other form of discrimination.

Age discrimination is closely related to stereotypes of ageing. Stereotypes are ideas held by some individuals about members of a particular group, based solely on membership of that group, in this case people who are older. In general, there are two broad but distinct views about ageing:

- Ageing is viewed as a time of opportunities and possibilities: an active, fluid, 'positive' image of old age.

- Ageing is viewed as a time of dependence, decline and disadvantage: a more passive, inevitable, 'negative' image of old age (Martin, 2006).

Both of these depictions represent stereotypes, in that the real experiences of older people are very diverse, and likely to range between these extremes. In negative stereotypes, older people are often caricatured as frail, forgetful, shabby, out of date and on the edge of senility and death (Featherstone and Hepworth, 2005). Images of mental and physical decline are all too common in both the literature and the media, and reflect the myth that they are an inevitable consequence of ageing (Kessler et al., 2004).

Positive stereotypes of ageing also assign broad attributes to older people, for example, that they are wise and experienced in life. However, such stereotypes can also be problematic as they imply that successful ageing is based on the following attributes:

- avoidance of disease and disability;
- high levels of physical and cognitive functioning;
- active engagement with life.

Holstein and Minkler (2003) argue that using the above criteria effectively relegates large sections of the older population to the 'unsuccessful' category, constituting an alternative form of ageism. Consequently, any form of stereotyping of older people has potential implications for mental health and well-being.

Participation in meaningful activity and mental health

All older people, including those with cognitive or physical frailty, have the potential to make a contribution to the society in which they live. Some will make this contribution largely within their own family, others through employment or voluntary work. Within the context of the family, more than one-third of older people are carers to ill and disabled people, while others provide childcare for relatives. It is important to recognise that the relationship between older people and their children, friends and neighbours is not one of simple dependency of old on young, but a complex exchange relationship that shifts only occasionally and gradually towards the younger people becoming the predominant care givers (Patterson, 2000).

In the UK, more than a million people over the age at which they are eligible to receive the state pension are in paid employment (Equal Opportunities Commission, 2005). Flexible forms of employment, such as self-employment and part-time working are enabling many older people to ease the transition from full-time employment to retirement (Platman, 2003). For some, this can provide a much needed supplement to pension income. For others the main motivation is the sense of worth and identity they gain from being employed (Social Exclusion Unit, 2006). There are many advantages for employers in hiring older workers, including reliability, prior investment in skills and know-how and company loyalty (Schultz, 2001). However, national (and international) trends in the employment of older workers show a decline in the economic participation of older people, and especially older men. Age discrimination within the workplace has been cited as a major contributing factor (Age Concern Policy Unit, 2006).

Volunteering can also play a significant role in people's lives as they move from work to retirement. Volunteering in later life has been associated with lower mortality and morbidity among volunteers (Harris and Thoresen, 2005; Lum and Lightfoot, 2005) as well as higher levels of well-being (Morrow-Howell et al., 2003). Studies have found that older volunteers are able to contribute even when they have chronic illness and functional difficulties themselves (Barron et al., 2006).

Even in advanced frailty, there are opportunities for older people to make a meaningful contribution to the communities in which they live. Taft et al. (2004), for example, describe the innovative use of oral history to provide residents of care homes with opportunities to share their knowledge and experience. Studies have found successful and positive caring experiences where care providers and older people formed friendships that provided mutual companionship and support (Roe et al., 2001).

Relationships and mental health

Repeated studies have found that older people nominate family relationships and contact with others as important determinants of their quality of life (Bowling, 2004). Older people who have strong social networks are happier and more likely to perceive themselves as healthy (Wenger and Tucker, 2002). Conversely, the absence of social relationships can lead to isolation and loneliness. Social relationships and support tend to be built up over a lifetime, and it is often difficult to begin to accumulate reserves in older age. Social isolation may be further increased as people get older by physical debility and lack of other reliable networks (Wenger and Tucker, 2002). Helping older people to develop and maintain connections with others in their community is therefore an effective nursing intervention for promoting mental well-being.

Relationships can also have a negative impact on mental health. For example, abusive relationships are linked to poor mental health, particularly for women (Age Concern, 2006). There is also evidence that caring relationships can have a negative impact on both physical and mental health, with those carers who provide high levels of physical care twice as likely to suffer ill health as non-carers (Carers UK, 2004).

The majority of older people continue to have close contact with family and friends. Data from the 2001 General Household Survey indicate that three-quarters of those aged 65 and over saw their relatives and friends weekly, and the majority saw their neighbours to chat to (Victor, 2006). It is estimated that around a third of the UK's adult population are grandparents, a role that is assuming increasing importance (Harper, 2005). However, increases in divorce and family separation can have a significant impact on grandparent–grandchildren relationships, and research has demonstrated the detrimental effect on grandparents' physical and emotional health when they lose contact with grandchildren (Drew and Smith, 1999).

Relationships have been found to be a particularly important component of well-being for older people who live in a care home. Recurrent themes within interview studies involving residents of care homes highlight the importance to relationships of continuity of staff, adequate communication, staff responsiveness, dependability and trust and a degree of personal control (Davies and Brown-Wilson, 2006).

Case study 2.1 offers a useful reflection.

Case study 2.1

Anne Porter is 81 years old and is being cared for in a residential home just 6 miles from the family home in the North of England. Anne, who trained as a primary-school teacher and practised until she was 60, has two sons, both of whom live over 50 miles away. Her husband Peter died 6 years ago. Anne was an active member of her community, involved in church activities and worked as a volunteer with a city-centre homeless project until she was 68. Anne had a stroke 4 years ago. The stroke occurred after a period of 18 months, when she experienced several Transient Ischaemic Attacks. This left Anne with severe hemiplegia down her left arm and leg. Attempts were made to enable Anne to remain in the family home, but her sons became concerned following a series of negative incidents involving community-based care services and suggested she move to the residential home. Anne was extremely reluctant.

Following a protracted 'settling in' period, Anne began to engage in some of the activities organised within the home, bingo, musical evenings and 'keep fit'. Lately, however, Anne has begun to lose interest in some of these. She is not sleeping well and does not seem to want to talk to others about how she is feeling. A suicide note has been found in her bedside table. The problem has been made worse by the fact that Mary, a care-worker at the home who got on well with Anne, retired 7 weeks ago.

Consider the following questions:
• What factors might contribute to Anne's apparent depression?
• What services might have helped Anne?
• How might the Care Home respond to Anne's changing situation?

Physical health

Physical health is generally seen as one of the key resources that older people bring to the experience of ageing, with older people themselves seeing the maintenance of physical and mental health and the avoidance of disability as important goals (Reed et al., 2004). Technological advances in health care and improved living conditions mean that many older people are living longer. However, these extra years are not always spent in good health. Perhaps not surprisingly, there is a close connection between physical and mental well-being, with higher levels of mental illness, particularly depression, among those with physical disabilities. Similarly, those with longstanding mental health conditions are also more likely to experience physical ill-health.

Many older people have at least one long-term condition affecting their physical health, such as arthritis or diabetes (Soule et al., 2005). The 2001 Census showed that the percentage of over 65s who report having a longstanding illness or chronic ill health was 60% for men and 65% for women (Soule et al., 2005). However, studies suggest that it is not the presence of a physical illness or disability per se that is the issue for older people, but its impact on their ability to 'go' and 'do' things (Reed et al., 2004). Current debates on the notion of 'successful ageing' caution against narrow definitions which exclude those with longstanding disabilities, in favour of models that view coping and adaptation as strategies for successful ageing (Holstein and Minkler, 2003). These are areas where expert nursing can be of particular help. However, this should not preclude us from recognising that poor physical health predisposes older people to poor mental health. The link between chronic pain and poor well-being, for instance, has been shown to exist in a number of research studies (Schofield et al., 2005). There are numerous situations where nursing interventions, such as offering regular pain relief, can alleviate physical symptoms, with subsequent benefits for mental well-being.

Poverty

Nearly two million older people in the UK live in poverty (defined as a household income less than 60% of the median income) (Age Concern, 2006). This is significant, since successive government reports have demonstrated a link between poverty and ill health (Department of Health and Social Security, 1980; Whitehead, 1988; Department of Health, 1998). In particular, mental illness is strongly associated with poverty; for example, people living in England and Wales in deprived industrial areas are more likely to be treated for depression than people living in any other type of area (Office for National Statistics, 2004).

The risk of poverty among older people in the UK is about three to four times higher than the typical risk of poverty in Europe (Burholt and Windle, 2006). Moreover, people aged 75 and over rely more on benefits as a source of income and receive a smaller proportion of their income from occupational pensions and investments than younger pensioners. A recent study in the UK explored the key determinants of poverty in old age (Burholt and Windle, 2006). The findings indicate that women, people living alone, people who are widowed, divorced or separated and people who are in poor health, have a lower education, and live in deprived neighbourhoods tend to have low levels of material resources and income in old age. These people are likely to be at particular risk of developing mental health conditions.

Transitions and the threat to mental health

For many people, later life consists of a series of changes or transitions. A transition can be defined as: 'The passage or movement from one state, condition or place to another' (Chick and Meleis, 1986, p. 237). The kinds of transition most commonly experienced by older people include changes within relationships, in employment status, in accommodation and in health and physical functioning. Some transitions can be planned, while others happen suddenly and without any opportunity to make preparations. There is now considerable research evidence to suggest that people undergoing transition tend to be more vulnerable to risks that may affect their health and well-being, including their mental health (Meleis et al., 2000). Transitions often require an individual to incorporate new knowledge and information and to alter their behaviour. As a result, their definition of 'self' may be threatened (Wilson, 1997; Meleis et al., 2000) and this can be particularly difficult for older people. The challenge for nurses and others involved in supporting individuals experiencing transition is to understand transition processes and to develop interventions which are effective in helping individuals to regain stability and a sense of well-being (Schumacher and Meleis, 1994).

Many older people have to cope with changes in their close relationships, often as a result of ill health or bereavement. Research carried out on behalf of Carers UK found that more than 1.5 million people over the age of 60 are providing unpaid care for a relative or friend (Buckler and Yeandle, 2005), with more than 8000 of these carers aged 90 and over, predominantly husbands caring for their wives. Older carers are often in poor health themselves and are more likely to have a limiting long-term illness. Older people in such situations may be at particular risk of mental health conditions. The loss of relationships through bereavement is also a common feature in later life. Although most people are able to cope with bereavement with the support of family and friends, some will experience a more complicated grief reaction, which can contribute to mental health conditions.

The onset of any mental health condition can also be seen as a time of transition, and this is particularly stressful, since there is usually a time of uncertainty prior to a diagnosis being reached. During this period, both family carer and care recipient can experience significant anxiety, as they will be unsure as to what they are facing (Farran et al., 2003). From the perspective of carers, changes in the behaviour of the older person with a mental health condition and uncertainty about the future are often the most difficult aspects to cope with.

People with severe mental health conditions, including dementia, may have difficulty in making and communicating decisions. Very few people are unable to be involved in making choices at all, but some may have partial or fluctuating mental capacity and may need help with communication. Pioneering work within the area of communication with older people with dementia has illustrated both the possibility and impact of supporting and training care staff in skilled communication practices, even with people whose verbal communication is limited (Allan, 2001). As the condition progresses, it is possible that the rewards from the relationship between the family carer and care recipient will diminish; for example, they may no longer be able to offer expressions of gratitude or recognition (Wuest et al., 2001), and this may contribute to depression on the part of the family carer (Williamson and Shaffer, 2001).

The significance of continuity

Psychosocial and sociological perspectives can help to broaden our understanding when thinking about potential strategies for working with older people with mental health needs and help us to provide effective support during major transition. Much of this work relies on notions of continuity in the lives of older people. Atchley (2000) draws upon notions of the internal and external self, and suggests that in order to maintain a successful, happy old age, every person needs to be supported to manage their own life within a generally consistent framework. Internally, people need to be allowed to make decisions in the way they always have. People also need to be able to maintain their self-esteem and integrity. Externally, individuals need to continue in positive roles, compensate for losses (physical and mental) and preserve social support and reciprocal relationships. If these external and internal elements of the self are disrupted, the likelihood, according to Atchley (2000), of poor self-image and unhappiness are heightened. Nilsson et al., (1998) draw on similar themes and suggest that feeling embedded within social networks, being meaningfully active, having links with the past and being able to continue to live a life which is consistent with personal beliefs all contribute to a successful old age. These themes are consistent with the findings of the review of mental health in later life discussed earlier (Age Concern, 2006). In particular, the significance of social relationships in maintaining good mental health for older people should not be underestimated. Godfrey and Denby (2004) list intimate relationships, the presence of a confidante, quality of ties and reciprocal relationships as important factors in preventing social isolation and risk of depression, both within care homes and in community settings.

Experiences of services

For many people with dementia and/or depression and their families, the prospect of using formal services can be daunting. Too often, services for older people with mental health needs are criticised for being inflexible, impersonal, institutional in form and unable to provide continuity. Where good-quality services, resourced by skilled staff, do exist, these tend to be local and small in scale, and there is a need to share models of good practice more widely. There is also continued evidence of ageism in the provision of mental health services with services for adults up to the age of 65 (adults of working age) configured separately to those for adults aged 65 and over (older people). Furthermore, a recent review suggested that those for older people are inferior (Healthcare Commission, 2006). There are also problems of access to mental health services in residential care settings; for example, research in care homes suggests that depression is often undiagnosed and treatments under-utilised.

The mental health needs of older people from black and minority ethnic communities have been particularly neglected. We know that there are lower levels of awareness of conditions such as depression and dementia within these groups and that older people and their families from black and minority ethnic communities have problems accessing help from services (Moriarty, 2005). There is insufficient evidence to date on whether integrated or separate services are more effective, but the need for more culturally appropriate and sensitive services is clear. Research carried out by the Policy Research Institute on Ageing and Ethnicity (2005) found that a lack of knowledge about services, language difficulties and the expectation on behalf of service providers that elders from black and minority ethnic groups will 'look after their own' are particular barriers to effective care.

It might be argued that current services have evolved out of a state-sponsored culture of dependency, whereby the image of the dependent, inactive older person has prevailed. Such service models have done little to alleviate the difficulties faced by older people with mental health needs, with some commentators arguing that these models and cultures actively promote poor mental health. The work of Kitwood (1997) is a case in point here. Kitwood argued that neurological impairment alone could not account for the changes experienced by the person with dementia and proposed that impairment and detrimental psychosocial aspects of the care environment conspire to 'strip' the individual with dementia of 'personhood'. This idea gives those working with people with dementia, particularly those in long-term care settings, a new lens from which to view practices and routines, and provides a framework within which professional behaviours, intentional or otherwise, might be related to disease progression, deterioration and disintegration of the self. Others, too, notably Sabat (2004), have endeavoured to analyse the nature of interactions, both within and outside care services which might undermine the status, confidence and self-identity of older people.

Community support: A model for the future

It is clear that the maintenance of home and family life plays an important role in helping to sustain continuity and prevent further difficulties for older people with organic or functional mental health conditions. The idea of long-term community-based support is therefore appealing. A growing number of such services have emerged for older people with dementia in recent years. These services, often providing support to both the person with dementia and their families for extended periods of time, have also been evaluated well from a number of perspectives. The focus of such developments is on building and sustaining relationships, flexible service provision, engaging people with dementia in meaningful activities and use of community or neighbourhood resources (Ryan et al., 2004). It is also felt that the intention of such services is not so much to prevent admission to care but rather to promote the idea of appropriate and timely admission to care.

An Audit Commission report in the UK (Audit Commission, 2000) was able to point to the following as being important advantages of the provision of specialist community-based services for older people with enduring mental health conditions:

- better understanding of the problems faced by older people and their families;
- greater continuity;
- greater coordination.

Other work around functional mental health difficulties has indicated moderate success for community-based provision in terms of reduction in symptoms. Van Citters and Bartels (2004) reviewed 17 experimental or quasi-experimental studies looking at the effectiveness of such provision in the USA. A range of models can be identified through this work, with an emphasis on multi-agency, case-intensive approaches towards people living in their own homes.

Case study 2.2 offers a useful reflection.

Case study 2.2

Eric and Patricia have lived in the same neighbourhood for almost 20 years. After spending time in the army doing his National Service, Eric returned home to work in a small factory. He retired 7 years ago. The couple have a son who lives 3 miles away and is married with three children. Five years ago, Eric began experiencing memory problems. Patricia became concerned and broached the subject with Eric. Reluctantly, he agreed to meet with his GP. A referral to a memory clinic was made and after several hospital visits Eric was diagnosed with Alzheimer's disease. The diagnosis had an immediate impact upon the lives of the couple. Both were dependent upon Eric doing all of the driving (shops, visits to see family and friends, trips into the countryside and so on). When he was told he could no longer do this, their participation in joint activities was immediately threatened. Eric felt he was not playing his part, a feeling which undermined his self-confidence. He became quiet and separate from the world. Despite her love for Eric, Patricia found things hard as the isolation began to impact upon their life as a couple. She felt she needed a break from Eric's 'forgetfulness' and increasing frustration at not being able to participate in social life. Eric finally agreed to go into a respite facility for a couple of weeks. The time apart was hard for both, Patricia felt guilty about leaving Eric for such a long time. Eric felt lonely and since his return Patricia feels that he has deteriorated significantly.

Consider the following questions:
- How has society contributed to Eric and Patricia's plight?
- What might have been put in place to help?

Conclusion

Mental health and older people's services have for many years been neglected by policy-makers and given low priority in resource allocation (Age Concern, 2006). However, there is now widespread recognition that this needs to change. The public health white paper 'Choosing Health' (Department of Health, 2004) stated that: 'Transforming the NHS from a sickness service to a health service is not just a matter of promoting physical health. Understanding how everyone in the NHS can promote mental well-being is equally important.'

Within this chapter, we hope that we have been able to provide some insights into how this important goal might be achieved. A useful starting-point is the recent Department of Health guidance in relation to the development of services, resources and skills which are aimed at addressing these challenges. The document, 'Everybody's Business' (Department of Health/Care Services Improvement Partnership, 2005) builds on those sections of the National Service Framework for Older People (Department of Health, 2001) relevant to mental health. Within recommendations made in relation to home-care services, the report calls for:

- a person-centred approach;
- skilled and knowledgeable staff;
- a move away from task completion towards supporting independence;
- service provision 7 days per week, 24 h a day;
- supporting the choice to stay at home;
- maintaining meaningful activities.

Within residential settings, there is emphasis upon the culture of care homes to move towards models that sustain continuity, despite the obvious physical transitions older people face. Recommendations suggest that the following should be priorities within these settings:

- use of biographical approaches to seeking out information about older people and their lives;
- maintenance of skills and interests;
- involvement of relatives and families and their continued participation in the provision of care;
- the need to meet a wide range of cultural and faith needs;
- developing skilled communication practice by staff.

Table 2.1 gives a summary of the knowledge and skills needed to work with older people who have mental health needs.

Our understanding of ways to promote positive mental health in old age and support older people with mental health needs is rapidly increasing. In order to make a difference to the health and well-being of older people in our society, we must make good use of this knowledge in our day-to-day practice. We hope that within this chapter, we have prompted you to think about the many things that contribute to mental well-being in later life and your role in influencing these factors.

Table 2.1 Summary of the knowledge and skills.

- Appreciates the social and psychosocial context of mental illness in old age
- Is aware of those factors that support mental-health and well-being
- Recognises factors that may be associated with poor mental-health
- Examines own attitudes to ageing
- Recognises and challenges ageism in others
- Understands the nature of transitions in later life
- Appreciates the limitations of existing services in meeting the mental-health needs of older adults
- Understands the importance of community-based services in meeting the mental health needs of older people and their families
- Recognises the characteristics of residential-care settings that support good mental-health care for older people

References

Age Concern (2005) *How Ageist is Britain?* London, Age Concern England.

Age Concern (2006) *Promoting Mental Health and Well-Being in Later Life.* London, Age Concern and the Mental Health Foundation.

Age Concern Policy Unit (2006) *The Age Agenda: Public Policy and Older People.* London, Age Concern.

Allan, K. (2001) *Communication and Consultation: Exploring Ways for Staff to Involve People with Dementia in Developing Services.* York, UK, Joseph Rowntree Foundation.

Atchley, R. (2000) A continuity theory of normal aging. In: *Aging and Everyday Life* (J. Gubriam and J. Holstein, eds). London, Blackwell, pp. 47–64.

Audit Commission (2000) *Forget Me Not: Mental Health Services for Older People.* London, Audit Commission.

Barron, J.S., Song, M. and Fried, L.P. (2006) The heterogeneity of older adults able to participate in high-intensity volunteering. *Journal of the American Geriatrics Society* **54** Supplement 4, S106.

Bowling, A. (2004) A taxonomy and overview of quality of life. In: *Models of Quality of Life: A Taxonomy, Overview and Systematic Review of the Literature* (J. Brown, A. Bowling and T. Flynn, eds). Sheffield, UK, European Forum on Population Ageing Research, pp. 6–77.

Buckler, L. and Yeandle, S. (2005) *Older Carers in the UK.* London, Carers National.

Burholt, V. and Windle, G. (2006) *The Material Resources and Well-Being of Older People.* York, UK, Joseph Rowntree Foundation.

Carers UK (2004) *In poor health: The Impact of Caring on Health.* London, Carers UK.

Chick, N. and Meleis, A.I. (1986) Transitions: a nursing concern. In: *Nursing Research Methodology: Issues and Implementation* (P.L. Chinn, ed.). Rockville, MD, Aspen, pp. 237–257.

Davies, S. and Brown-Wilson, C. (2006) Creating community within care homes. In: *My Home Life: Quality of Life in Care Homes.* London, Help the Aged and the National Care Home Research and Development Forum, pp. 65–84.

Department of Health (1998) *Independent Inquiry into Inequalities in Health Report (Chair Sir Donald Acheson).* London, The Stationery Office.

Department of Health (2001) *National Service Framework for Older People.* London, The Stationery Office.

Department of Health (2004) *Choosing Health: Making Healthy Choices Easier.* London, The Stationery Office.

Department of Health and Social Security (1980) *The Black Report on Inequalities in Health.* London, HMSO.

Department of Health/Care Services Improvement Partnership (2005) *Everybody's Business. Integrated Mental Health Services for Older Adults: a Service Development Guide.* London, Department of Health.

Drew, L.M. and Smith, P.K. (1999) The impact of parental separation/divorce on grand-parent/grandchild relationships. *International Journal of Aging and Human Development* **48**, 191–215.

Equal Opportunities Commission (2005) *Pensions fact sheet.* http://www.eco.org.uk

Farran, C.J., Loukissa, D., Perraud, S. and Paun, O. (2003) Alzheimer's disease caregiving information and skills. Part I: care recipient issues and concerns. *Research in Nursing and Health* **26** (5), 366–75.

Featherstone, M. and Hepworth, M. (2005) Images of ageing: cultural representations of later life. In: *The Cambridge Handbook of Age and Ageing* (M. Johnson, ed.). Cambridge, Cambridge University Press, pp. 354–362.

Ferguson, C. and Keady, J. (2001) The mental health needs of older people and their carers: exploring tensions and new directions. In: *Working with Older People and their Families: Key Issues in Policy and Practice* (M. Nolan, S. Davies and G. Grant, eds). Buckingham, UK, Open University Press, pp. 120–138.

Godfrey, M. and Denby, T. (2004) *Depression and Older People: Towards Securing Well-Being in Later Life.* Bristol, UK, The Policy Press.

Harper, S. (2005) Grandparenthood. In: *The Cambridge Handbook of Age and Ageing* (M. Johnson, ed.). Cambridge, Cambridge University Press, pp. 422–428.

Harris A.H.S. and Thoresen C.E. (2005) Volunteering is associated with delayed mortality in older people: analysis of the Longitudinal Study of Aging. *Journal of Health Psychology* **10** (6), 739–752.

Healthcare Commission (2006) Living Well in Later Life: A Review of Progress against the National Service Framework for Older People. (Joint Report of The Healthcare Commission, The Audit Commission and The Commission for Social Care Inspection). London, Healthcare Commission.

Holstein, M.B. and Minkler, M. (2003) Self, society and the new gerontology. *The Gerontologist* **43** (6), 797–796.

Insel, K. and Badger, T. (2002) Deciphering the 4 D's: cognitive decline, delirium, depression and dementia – a review. *Journal of Advanced Nursing* **38** (4), 360–368.

Kessler, E., Racoczy, K. and Staudinger, U.M. (2004) The portrayal of older people in prime time television series: the mismatch with gerontological evidence. *Ageing and Society* 24: 531–552.

Kitwood, T. (1997) *Dementia Reconsidered: The Person Comes First.* Milton Keynes, UK, Open University Press.

Lum, T.Y. and Lightfoot, E. (2005) The effects of volunteering on the physical and mental health of older people. *Research on Aging* **27** (1), 31–55.

Manthorpe, J. and Iliffe, S. (2006) Anxiety and Depression. *Nursing Older People* **18** (1), 24–29.

Martin, W. (2006) Age, ageing and the body in everyday life. Paper given at the Agenet workshop, Brave new world: ageing research at Reading University, 3 July. http://www.fp.rdg.ac.uk/AGEnet/PreviousMeetings/June2006/Martin.pdf

Meleis, A.I., Sawyer, L.M., Im, E., Hilfinger Messias, D.K. and Schumacher, K. (2000) Experiencing transitions: an emerging middle-range theory. *Advances in Nursing Science* **23** (1), 12–28.

Melzer, D., Ely, M. and Brayne, C. (1997) Cognitive impairment in elderly people: population based estimate of the future in England, Scotland and Wales. *British Medical Journal* 315, 462.

Moriarty, J. (2005) *Update for SCIE Best Practice Guide on Assessing the Mental Health Needs of Older People*. London, Social Care Workforce Research Unit, Kings College.

Morrow-Howell, N., Hinterlong, J., Rozario, P.A. and Tang, F. (2003) Effects of volunteering on the well-being of older adults. *The Journals of Gerontology Series B: Psychological Sciences and Social Sciences* **58**, S137–S145.

Nilsson, M., Ekman, S. and Sarvimäki, A. (1998) Ageing with joy or resigning to old age: older people's experiences of the quality of life in old age. *Health Care in Later Life* **3** (2), 94–110.

Office for National Statistics (2004) *The Varied Lives of Our Older People*. London, Office for National Statistics

Patterson, L. (2000) The tide is not rising. *Health Matters* **40** (1), 10–11.

Platman, K. (2003) The self-designed career in later life: a study of older portfolio workers in the United Kingdom. *Ageing and Society* **23** (3), 281–302.

Policy Research Institute on Ageing and Ethnicity (2005) *Minority elderly health and social care in the United Kingdom*. Research briefing. http://www.priae.org.uk

Reed, J., Stanley, C. and Clarke, C. (2004) *Health, Well-Being and Older People*. Bristol, UK, The Policy Press.

Roe, B., Whattam, M., Young, H. and Dimond, M. (2001) Elders' perceptions of formal and informal care: aspects of getting and receiving help for their activities of daily living. *Journal of Clinical Nursing* **10** (3), 398–405.

Ryan, T., Nolan, M., Enderby, P. and Reid, D. (2004) 'Part of the Family': Sources of satisfaction amongst a group of community-based dementia care workers. *Health and Social Care in the Community* **12** (2), 111–118.

Sabat, S. (2004) *The Experience of Alzheimer's Disease: Life through a Tangled Veil*. Oxford, Blackwell Publishing.

Schofield, P., Dunham, M., Clarke, A., Faulkner, M., Ryan, T. and Howarth, A. (2005) *An Annotated Bibliography for the Management of Pain in the Older Adult*. Sheffield, UK, University of Sheffield.

Schultz, J.H. (2001) Productive aging: an economist's views. In *Productive Aging: Concepts and Challenges*. Sherraden, M.W., Hinterlong, J., Morrow-Howell, N. eds). Baltimore, John Hopkins University Press, pp. 145–174.

Schumacher, K.L. and Meleis, A.I. (1994) Transitions: a central concept in nursing. *Journal of Nursing Scholarship* **26** (2), 119–27.

Social Exclusion Unit (2006) *A Sure Start to Later Life: Ending Inequalities for Older People*. London, Social Exclusion Unit.

Soule, A., Babb, P., Evandrou, M., Balchin, S. and Zealey, L. (2005) *Focus on Older People*. London, Office for National Statistics.

Taft, L., Stolder, M.E., Knutson, A.B., Tamke, K., Platt, J. and Bowlds, T. (2004) Oral history: Validating contributions of elders. *Geriatric Nursing* **25** (1), 38–43.

Van Citters, A. and Bartels, S. (2004) A systematic review of the effectiveness of community based mental health outreach services for older adults. *Psychiatric Services* **55** (11), 1237–1249.

Victor, C. (2006) Demographic and epidemiological trends in ageing. In: *Nursing Older People* (S. Redfern and F. Ross, eds). Edinburgh, Elsevier, pp. 23–28.

Wenger, G.C. and Tucker, I. (2002) Using network variation in practice: identification of support network type. *Health and Social Care in the Community* **10** (1), 28–35.

Wuest, J., Ericson, P.K., Stern, P.N. and Irwin, G.W. (2001) Connected and disconnected support: the impact on the caregiving process in Alzheimer's disease. *Health Care for Women International* **22** (1/2), 115–130.

Whitehead, M. (1988) *The Health Divide.* London, Pelican.

Williamson, G.M. and Shaffer, D.R. (2001) The family relationships in late life project relationship quality and potentially harmful behaviours by spousal caregivers: How we were then, how we are now. *Psychology and Aging* **16** (2), 217–226.

Wilson, S.A. (1997) The transition to nursing home life: a comparison of planned and unplanned admissions. *Journal of Advanced Nursing* **26** (5), 864–871.

Chapter 3
Normal Physiological Ageing

Roger Watson

Introduction

This chapter will consider how the process of ageing affects the brain. The process of biological ageing in the human body is indisputable and inevitable. The outward signs of ageing, despite our best efforts to mask them, are obvious, especially the skin and hair. These signs of ageing are superficial and relatively unimportant compared with the changes in the other organ systems in the body. While it is well established that ageing and disease are not necessarily synonymous, it is clear that there is a relationship between ageing and disease and, indeed, between ageing and disability (Tinker, 1997). If there were no such link – if we all lived perfectly healthy lives from birth to death without a particular pattern of diseases in old age – there would be little interest in the ageing process. Every organ of the body changes as we age, including the brain, and these changes mean that efficiency declines.

One of the major problems in gerontology is in deciding what is normal and what is abnormal (Watson, 2006). This question is very hard to answer. Clearly, taking the skeletomuscular system as an example, being able to walk without impairment due to pain or stiffness of joints, in old age, could be considered to be normal, and being completely immobile could be considered to be abnormal. However, the skeletomuscular system declines with age: the muscles atrophy, the tendons and ligaments become less flexible, and the bones lose calcium (Watson, 2006); there is bound to be some decline in performance, and the normal range of performance will be less than that for younger people. However, the point at which 'normal' gerontological changes become 'abnormal' and fall within the domain of geriatric medicine is not clear. The same principles apply to any organ system of the body, including the brain.

This chapter, therefore, is focused on the normal changes that take place with ageing in the brain, but due to the blurred boundaries between normal and abnormal, the material will extend into some of the abnormal aspects to illustrate how the ageing of the brain can become a problem for some people.

The process of ageing

There are various theories of ageing including the genetic, the cellular and the physiological. However, precisely why we age and how we age is not fully understood. From an evolutionary perspective, it can be considered that we age because our bodies exist to carry and exchange gametes – eggs and sperm which do not age – but that the body itself is disposable (the disposable soma theory) (Kirkwood, 2000). The actual mechanism of ageing seems to lie at the genetic level – while having a profound effect at the cellular and physiological level – in that there is an accumulation of faults in the replication of genes throughout life leading to faults in the synthesis of proteins which control every aspect of our lives. The longer we live, the greater the number of faults we accumulate until this becomes incompatible with survival (Kirkwood, 2002).

The origin of the faults at the genetic level is oxygen. Oxygen, while being essential for our survival, is highly toxic and we are designed to survive through a range of biochemical mechanisms which help to neutralise this threat and also to repair most of the damage that is done to our genes (Kirkwood, 2002). However, as we age, the survival and repair mechanisms become less efficient, faults accumulate and ageing takes place. All the organs and systems of the body, including the brain, are subject to this ageing process.

The ageing brain

The ageing of the brain can be approached from the neurobiological, psychological or functional perspectives. From the neurobiological perspective, there are two considerations: the anatomical and the neurochemical. As we age, the size of the brain declines (Rabbitt, 2005), the mass of the brain tissue reduces, while the ventricles, containing cerebrospinal fluid which bathes and cushions the brain, enlarge. This is particularly marked in the brains of people who have developed Alzheimer's disease but is progressive throughout normal ageing and in people who have not developed Alzheimer's disease. The changes in the neurochemicals in the brain, such as dopamine and noradrenaline – also known as neurotransmitters – are complicated, but as a general principle, the pathways in which these neurochemicals work become less responsive to the stimuli of the neurochemicals which act to transmit signals chemically between nerve cells (Baltes et al., 2005). The speed of conduction along the nerve cells in the brain – the neurons – becomes slower with age (Watson, 2006). However, the sum total of these changes, which are common to everyone as they age, is not significant, and stereotypes of older people losing their memory, being unable to keep up intellectually with younger people and generally losing their mental faculties should be dismissed. The changes, while measurable, are set against a background of considerable reserve mental capacity and the ability to compensate for such changes; admittedly, the reserve capacity itself declines with age (Mori et al., 1997), but, for the normal lifespan and even into advanced old age, the function of the brain is sufficient to maintain a normal – for that person – and independent life.

The psychological approaches to ageing include such things as cognitive function, intelligence, memory and personality, and these take a mainly psycho-metric approach using standardised instruments to assess the various aspects of the function of the brain. Intelligence is one measure of mental ability and is related to such things as performance in examinations and passing various tests. It is composed of different aspects such as problem-solving and visual-spatial ability. Essentially, however, intelligence is composed of fluid intelligence and crystallised intelligence (Sternberg and Grigorenko, 2005); the former is con-cerned with rapid problem-solving 'on the spot' ability unrelated to former learning, while the latter is more related to problem-solving based on learning. Crystallised intelligence is often considered to be analogous to wisdom. Scores on intelligence tests are composed of scores for both fluid and crystallised intel-ligence, while both can be measured separately. It has been demonstrated that in advanced old age, in the absence of disease that would adversely affect cog-nitive function, overall intelligence does not change (Sternberg and Grigorenko, 2005). However, it has also been demonstrated that the two components to intelligence change differently with age: fluid intelligence declines with age, while crystallised remains stable or even continues to increase (Sternberg and Grigorenko, 2005). The overall effect is that young and old people can be equally good at solving problems but will do so in different ways.

Memory is adversely affected by ageing, and it is not uncommon for people, as they get older, to complain that their memory is not as good as it used to be. There is also a stereotyped view of older people being able to recall events from the past very clearly but unable to remember things that have happened very recently. However, there is some truth to the above. Memory is composed of three components: sensory memory, short-term memory and long-term mem-ory (Maylor, 2005). Sensory memory is the means by which we sense events, e.g. conversations, facts and faces, that can be memorised. Clearly, not everything that we sense is remembered; if it were, we would become saturated with infor-mation and overloaded with memories. Therefore, sensory memory is selective. Short-term memory is used to store information that is important to us before it is either forgotten or stored permanently in our long-term memory. Our short-term memory can hold between five and nine pieces of information at any time, and the information in the short-term memory can be displaced by adding new pieces of information. If you try to memorise a list of facts, it becomes harder the more facts that are added, and you reach a point where you try to exclude new facts so that you may remember those you have recalled. Long-term memory is a permanent store of information which is transferred from the short-term memory. Not everything that is held in the short-term memory is stored in the short-term memory; the mechanisms by which information becomes stored in the long-term memory are not fully understood, but rehearsal is part of it; repeatedly trying to keep facts in your short-term memory helps to get those facts into your long-term memory (Maylor, 2005). This is what lies behind the practice of studying for an exam: you read and reread a series of facts until, at some point, you are sure that they are in your long-term memory. This is then tested in an examination. Obviously, some people are better at memorising facts than others; these people can either hold more information in their short-term memory or transfer more information to their long-term memory. Different people have different strategies for learning material and storing it in their long-term memory and undertaking a prolonged period of study, such as a university-degree programme, usually helps people to find out how best they learn.

Ageing appears to affect the short-term memory (Maylor, 2005). Other than in pathological conditions, such as Alzheimer's disease, sensory and long-term memory do not appear to be adversely affected by age. Therefore, there is some truth in the stereotype of older people who can recall, vividly, events in the past but who do have problems remembering what happened very recently. However, this is not usually a problem because there are many ways in which we can compensate – and do compensate – for a failing short-term memory. Short-term memory is not just a problem for older people; as already explained, we can hold only a limited amount of information in our short-term memory at any age, and as we grow busier, we are dependent upon keeping a note of our appointments and engagements. This is to compensate for our limited short-term memory: throughout the course of a day, many things will happen that we are required to remember, but we know that we will not remember them all, and we take a note often in a diary. Older people can use diaries, post-its and other notes to help their memory if they are having difficulty. An older person may become distressed at a failing memory but should be reassured that, within limits, this is perfectly normal and that they can do something about it. On the other hand, there is a syndrome called age-associated memory impairment (AAMI) (Deary, 1995), which is not considered to be normal and which causes some older people significant problems. The cardinal feature of AAMI is a decline in memory function which is greater than one standard deviation below the mean for memory performance and that, in statistical terms means that is outside a normal range of ability. Which can be measured using a tachistoscope – a device for projecting images and testing the ability to memorise them. The person must have had no problems with cognitive function prior to AAMI and not diagnosed with dementia. However, the real sign of AAMI is functional: the person suffering from AAMI has loss of memory which severely affects their daily life. The person with AAMI can still function but will have major lapses of memory; appointments will be forgotten and it may be that they will drive to the shops and, on leaving the shop, have no idea where they parked their car, for example. It is unclear whether or not AAMI is a necessary prelude to severe cognitive decline and dementia or whether it is a separate phenomenon (Deary, 1995). Clearly, some people with AAMI will proceed to develop dementia. Help is available for AAMI, as it is for people with dementia, at memory clinics (Passmore and Craig, 2004) where a range of advice is offered on how to try to compensate for loss of memory, safety around the home and advice about finances. There is some evidence that drug treatment including the use of nicotine patches may be of benefit in AAMI (White and Levin, 2004).

In addition to changes in memory as we age, attention changes in that it becomes more difficult to attend to relevant information and to inhibit irrelevant information (Baltes et al., 2005). Clearly, there will be some interaction here with memory; if it becomes harder to sort out what is relevant from what is irrelevant, then it will be harder to know what it is important to remember. This means that an older person will become more easily distracted when they are trying to absorb information – but it does not mean that they are incapable of absorbing information. The right circumstances need to be created, for example, if a health professional is going to explain to older persons their diagnosis and any treatment, such as medication, that they are going to receive. A busy hospital ward or waiting area is not ideal, as there may be too many distractions. Older persons, just like any other person, may not admit to not understanding or absorbing what they have been told, or they may misapprehend and depart with the wrong information. In either case, it is the responsibility of the health professional to make sure that the situation is right for information to be understood (Watson, 2006), and the level of understanding can be checked by appropriate questions. In the same vein, it is worth considering the senses, especially vision and hearing (Magrain and Boulton, 2005). While not strictly speaking of the brain, these systems are affected by ageing, and this will have an adverse effect of the extent and quality of information reaching the brain. As we age, both vision and hearing decline, but this is not a consequence of changes to the nervous system. Vision declines because of changes in the shape of the lens in the eye. The lens is responsible for focusing images on the retina – the part of the eye that senses light – and the point in the eye at which the image is focused changes as the shape of the lens changes. As we age, the ability to focus on the retina declines, and typically, we become more 'long-sighted'. However, this change is easily corrected by wearing spectacles, and, while spectacles are worn by younger people, they are more commonly worn by older people, and it is very uncommon for an older person not to wear spectacles, at least for reading. The eye changes in other ways as we age but the most profound of these is a thickening and opacity of the lens of the eye (Magrain and Boulton, 2005). This is common to all older people but, in an advanced state, is known as cataract. Cataract reduces the quality of vision by narrowing the visual field and reducing the clarity of what is viewed. Cataract can be corrected by surgery, but it is probably true to say that if each of us lived long enough, we would, eventually, develop cataract. Similarly, if each of us lived long enough, we would become very hard of hearing, if not hearing-impaired, because this is another inevitable aspect of ageing. There are several factors such as increased cerumen (ear wax) accumulation – easily remedied – but the main factor is reduced efficiency of the system of small bones that transmit sound from the outer to the inner ear (Magrain and Boulton, 2005). This system of small bones – the maleus, incus and stapes – need to articulate freely to transmit sound most efficiently, but as we age, they gradually become fused together, and this transmits sound less efficiently from the outer to the inner ear.

While the loss of hearing and vision is not a direct result of any ageing changes in the brain itself, the deterioration of these sense organs, which provide information to the brain, can have a profound effect on function. At its worst, it can lead to sensory deprivation, which will have adverse effects on the brain and can lead to isolation and confusion (Rabbitt, 2005). At a more practical level, a decline in both hearing and vision will have a detrimental effect of the extent to which an older person may understand information, and this may lead people, such as health workers, to conclude that there is something wrong with an older person's understanding as such. Knowledge of the deteriorating senses with ageing will ensure that health professionals take time with older people to ensure that they have understood information (Watson, 2006). This process can be helped by ensuring that older people are addressed directly and clearly – without shouting – and that any written information, especially where health and safety are concerned as with prescribed drugs, is written clearly using large, bold and easy-to-read fonts (Watson, 2006).

The remaining senses, smell, taste and touch, also decline with age, and this also has implications for the transmission of information to the brain. It must not be assumed that older people cannot feel pain or heat and cold, but they do have slightly increased pain thresholds and find it less easy to locate and describe pain. Again, this is not a result of decline in brain function, rather a decline in the quality of the information reaching the brain. In the case of smell and taste – and smell is a major component of the way in which we taste food – older people do frequently complain that they lose their taste for food and, as a result, may add increasing quantities of sugar or salt to sweet and savoury foods, respectively, to enhance the taste. Clearly, this may be detrimental to health, especially higher levels of salt, and its effect on the cardiovascular system and dietetic advice may be necessary to help an older person choose foods that they like and that are more 'tasty' such as curries and pasta sauces – if the older person likes to eat such foods.

Latent potential

In common with most systems of the body, we do not use the nervous system, of which the brain is the key component, to the full. For example, most of the time, we only us about 10% of the capacity of the heart and lungs as we go about our daily lives. However, if we need to – for example, running to catch a bus – then we can use a much greater percentage of the capacity. This is called latent potential, and the brain, likewise, has latent potential; if necessary, we can call on greater reserves of potential in the brain, and this partly protects us against the effects of ageing (Baltes et al., 2005). The function of the brain declines as we age across a range of functions, but we can call on latent potential to compensate.

However, it appears that latent potential also declines with ageing, meaning that compensation is only possible up to a point (Baltes et al., 2005).

Cognitive function

Some aspects of cognitive function have already been referred to, but this section will consider the severe decline in cognitive function that can occur with ageing, leading to dementia. This chapter is about normal aspects of the ageing brain, but as with all aspects of gerontology, it is extremely hard to say where normal ageing ends and abnormal ageing begins. This was exemplified earlier using the skeltomuscular system as an example, but this equally applies to the brain. As described, some decline in the function of the brain in terms of memory, attention span and distraction take place with ageing, and some people, who are not diagnosed with dementia, do display AAMI, which has an adverse effect on their daily life. However, possibly excluding AAMI, older people can function independently, and any effects of the ageing brain are either minimal or negligible. At the other end of the cognitive spectrum, however, some older people display a severe loss of cognitive function, leading to dementia and loss of independence, and this is not reversible. Such a severe loss of cognitive function is not considered to be normal; however, the association between ageing and dementia is very strong. Figures available from the Alzheimer's Society (www.alzheimers.org.uk) show that, from the age of 65 onwards, the prevalence of dementia increases to the point where one in two people over the age of 90 will have some degree of dementia. The question remains, therefore, whether or not dementia is an inevitable part of the ageing process, and, if we all lived sufficiently long, would we all, ultimately, develop dementia? The question is also raised of whether or not the mild cognitive changes associated with ageing, the phenomenon of AAMI, and dementia are, in fact, a continuum. For this reason, it is appropriate to consider dementia in a chapter on normal ageing, as some of the changes associated with dementia can be found in all ageing brains.

Dementia, of course, is a diagnosis; it results from several causes, but the principal causes are Alzheimer's disease, cerebrovascular disease and Lewy body disease (Woods, 2005). These are all distinct phenomena but are similar in that they all lead to severe loss of function of regions of the brain. While the ageing brain naturally diminishes in size, Alzheimer's disease leads to a severe reduction in the size of the brain, especially the temporal lobes, but is also characterised by specific markers in the brain, areas of devastation called neurofibrillary plaques and tangles (Woods, 2005). Cerebrovascular disease, arising due to atherosclerosis of the vascular system of the brain, leads to deprivation of the blood supply to areas of the brain and subsequent loss of brain tissue. Atherosclerosis is another normal aspect of ageing that affects the whole of the cardiovascular system (Tian, 2005). In the brain, it has other effects such as stroke, mini-strokes and transient ischaemic attacks. However, while recovery is possible from the above, cerebrovascular disease leading to dementia is irreversible. Lewy body dementia, sometimes associated with Parkinson's disease, arises from the accumulation of Lewy bodies in the brain (Woods, 2005). Lewy bodies are round deposits of damaged neurons in the brain, and the disease is very similar to Alzheimer's disease, only being afforded a separate diagnosis in recent years.

The dilemma about whether or not dementia is a normal part of the ageing process arises because many of the features of the dementias mentioned above appear to be part of the normal process of ageing. For example, neurofibrillary plaques and tangles can be found in the brains of people who have not been diagnosed with dementia (Watson, 1992), as can Lewy bodies. Cerebrovascular disease is part of the normal ageing process and will be found, to some extent, in all ageing brains. There seems to be no doubt that the features of the dementias mentioned above are associated with severe and irreversible cognitive decline; they are not simply artefacts or do not correlate with these diseases. However, the question remains as to why some people with these features display no cognitive decline, and others do: is there a continuum from normal cognitive function in younger years to declining cognitive function with age, with this process taking place faster in some individuals than in others? Alternatively, are these conditions abnormal with their own pathology and resulting in cognitive decline which is not inevitable, no matter how many years a person lives for? There is no answer to the above questions, but they raise scientific possibilities and also philosophical questions. The scientific possibilities, if the dementias are discrete and abnormal, age-correlated, but not caused by ageing, include the possibility of curing, slowing down or preventing these conditions. On the other hand, if the dementias are an inevitable part of the ageing process and can be alleviated, as described above, then the possibility exists of slowing down or even reversing the effects of ageing on the brain (Watson, 1992). Drug therapies are available for dementia, but they do not offer the possibility of cure at the moment, and the extent to which they slow down the process seems to be related to the extent to which therapy is provided in the early stages (NICE, 2001).

Conclusion

As the body ages, so does the brain. While the outward manifestations of ageing are more obvious and predictable, the effects of ageing on the brain are less obvious and, to some extent, less predictable. Ageing has consequences for all aspects of cognitive ability: intelligence, memory and the ability to process information. However, the effects of ageing on the brain are greater for some individuals than others, and even when the effects of ageing on the brain are manifest, this does not mean that the older person is incapable of leading an active life and participating in decision-making. This chapter has reviewed some of the physiological effects of ageing on the brain and, thereby, on the lives of some older people. The implications of caring for older people in whom the effects of ageing in the brain are manifest are a challenge for the caring professions, and the essence of good care is to assess each person on an individual basis.

References

Baltes, P.B., Freund, A.M. and Li, S-C. (2005) The psychological science of human ageing. In: *The Cambridge Handbook of Age and Ageing* (M.L. Johnson, ed.). Cambridge, Cambridge University Press, pp. 47–71.

Deary, I.J. (1995) Age-associated memory impairment: a suitable case for treatment. *Ageing and Society* **15**, 393–406.

Kirkwood, T. (2000) *Time of Our Lives*. London, Weidenfeld & Nicolson.

Kirkwood, T. (2002) Evolution of ageing. *Mechanisms of Ageing and Development* **123**, 737–745.

Magrain, T.H. and Boulton, M. (2005) Sensory impairment. In: *The Cambridge Handbook of Age and Ageing* (M.L. Johnson, ed.). Cambridge, Cambridge University Press, pp. 121–130.

Maylor, E.A. (2005) Age-related changes in memory. In: *The Cambridge Handbook of Age and Ageing* (M.L. Johnson, ed.). Cambridge, Cambridge University Press, pp. 200–208.

Mori, E., Hirono, N., Yamashita, H., Imamura, T., Ikejiri, Y., Ikeda, M., Kitagaki, H., Shimomura, T. and Yoneda, Y. (1997) Premorbid brain size as a determinant of reserve capacity against intellectual decline in Alzheimer's disease *American Journal of Psychiatry* **154**, 18–24.

NICE (National Institute for Health and Clinical Excellence) (2001) *Guidance on the Use of Donepezil (Aricept), Rivastigmine (Exelon) and Galantamine (Reminyl) for the Treatment of Alzheimer's Disease*. London, NICE.

Passmore, A.P. and Craig, D.A. (2004) The future of memory clinics. *Psychiatric Bulletin* **28**, 375–377.

Rabbitt, P. (2005) Cognitive changes across the lifespan. In: *The Cambridge Handbook of Age and Ageing* (M.L. Johnson, ed.). Cambridge, Cambridge University Press, pp. 190–199.

Sternberg, R.J. and Grigorenko, E.L. (2005) Intelligence and wisdom. In: *The Cambridge Handbook of Age and Ageing* (M.L. Johnson, ed.), Cambridge, Cambridge University Press, pp. 209–215.

Tian, J. (2005) Dementia in an Asian context. In: *The Cambridge Handbook of Age and Ageing* (M.L. Johnson, ed.). Cambridge, Cambridge University Press, pp. 261–272.

Tinker, A. (1997) *Older People in Modern Society*. London, Longman.

Watson, R. (1992) Alzheimer's disease: does it exist? *Nursing Standard* **6** (43), 29–31.

Watson, R. (2006) Care of older people. In *Nursing Practice: Hospital and Home: the Adult* (M. Alexander, T. Fawcett, and P. Runciman, eds). Edinburgh, Elsevier, pp. 1131–1146.

White, H.K. and Levin, E.D. (2004) Chronic transdermal nicotine patch treatment effects on cognitive performance in age-associated memory impairment. *Psychopharmacology* **171**, 465–471

Woods, B. (2005) Dementia. In: *The Cambridge Handbook of Age and Ageing* (M.L. Johnson, ed.). Cambridge, Cambridge University Press, pp. 252–260.

Chapter 4
Values Underpinning Help, Support and Care

Jan Dewing

Introduction

Values and beliefs are the bedrock of nursing practice and influence how we work with and care about older people and their families. Surprisingly, given their influence, they are not always talked about in detail, as if there is some reticence or embarrassment about standing up and voicing our values. This chapter aims to have a discussion about the place and contribution values make in mental health and older people's nursing. In this chapter, I aim to establish that as a professional nurse, having values and knowing exactly what they are, matters. In particular, working out and clarifying our values, especially about ageing, is vital for nursing practice. Then, I will suggest that there is considerable commitment needed to ensure that our values are translated into actions and those actions are consistent with our values in the complex world of practice, where the values of person-centredness often seem to clash with the growing risk-aversion culture in health and social care for older people.

Values and beliefs

Values are a collection of ideas about the worth or importance of people, concepts or 'things'. They come from a person's beliefs. McCormack (2005, p. 44) says that beliefs are attitudes or dispositions about what is good, right, desirable or worthwhile. But more than this, beliefs are convictions that a person holds to be true. Beliefs are often held regardless of facts or truths. Beliefs need to be strongly held to enable us to achieve things – to motivate us. But beliefs that are too weak or too strong can sometimes lead to difficulties in life and work. Often, the consequences of strongly or weakly held beliefs can be seen in some individuals within mental health practice.

Values are beliefs that have become ordered into a (value) system with some sense of priorities or weighting. We have values about all sorts of things; for example, we have personal values, cultural values, social values and work values.

As way of illustration, Ludwick and Cipriano-Silva (2000) set out six tips concerned with working on cultural values:

- Recognise that values and beliefs vary not only among different cultures but also within cultures.
- View values and beliefs from different cultures within historical, health care, cultural, spiritual and religious contexts.
- Learn as much as you can about the language, customs, beliefs and values of cultural groups, especially those with which you have the most contact.
- Be aware of your own cultural values and biases, a major step to decreasing ethnocentrism and cultural imposition. (A questionnaire on this can be found in Andrews and Herberg, 1999.)
- Be alert to and try to understand the non-verbal communications of your own and various cultures such as personal space preferences, body language and style of hair and clothing.
- Be aware of biocultural differences manifested in types of illness, in response to drugs and in health care practices (Ludwick and and Cipriano-Silva, 2000).

Values are everywhere

Ghaye (2005, p. 126) suggests that values are everywhere, and they matter. He also says that mattering about them matters, too. In nursing and other areas of health and social care, we can see that effective leaders work from a clear values and belief base which they openly share with others. Within each category or grouping of the beliefs we have, we value some things more than others. For example, while I believe in a healthy lifestyle, I may value not smoking at all more than not drinking too much at certain times. Thus, at times, either to ourselves or to others, our values and beliefs may appear incompatible. (See Table 4.1 for a framework that can enable you to work out your values.)

Table 4.1 Knowing your value systems

Personal values	Cultural values	Social values	Work values
E.g. compassion	E.g. diversity	E.g. free health care and education	E.g. stimulating, working in a team

Although values and beliefs tend to remain constant during our lives, we can have experiences whereby they become modified or even, on occasions, are significantly altered through a major life event or experience. In terms of nursing practice, it is helpful to recognise that many experiences in nursing can mean that our values and beliefs about person's, health, nursing and the world can be challenged and indeed may need to be challenged, if continuous attention to improving expertise in nursing older people is to be a central part of nursing practice. Challenge is not a one-off event or something that is offered only to a student for one module or as part of a practice experience, but instead it is better thought of as something that all nurses committed to life-long learning return to many times over the course of their working life. Committing to developing skills through structured reflection and supervision can help this process.

Personal and professional values

There is an interrelationship between personal and professional values. All nurses bring their personal values and beliefs with them into their work in some way. There are two approaches to this. The first argues that the personal and professional are separate. Thus, personal values and beliefs should be left at home. The other approach says persons cannot separate themselves from their values and beliefs. Values form part of what is sometimes referred to as personal or tacit knowledge (Higgs and Andresen 2001, p. 16), so nurses need to be actively reflecting on them and how they influence ways of working in health care. Given that working with older people with mental health needs often produces situations where values and beliefs can be core to decision-making, care planning and care delivery, it seems reasonable to argue that the second approach has more relevance to professional nursing practice.

Case study 4.1

Tom believed older people 'suffering' with dementia were vulnerable and needed to be kept as safe as possible. He also believed that older people with dementia were unable to make decisions for themselves.

Case study 4.2

Claire believed that older people with dementia were survivors and needed to have as much freedom as possible. She also believed that older people with dementia were generally able to make decisions for themselves well into the dementia process.

We can begin to imagine how both Tom and Claire's beliefs would influence how they worked within a team and how they cared for and nursed clients or patients on a day-to-day basis. It is worthwhile considering just how far reaching the impact of our values and beliefs spreads in day-to-day practice. To give you some idea of this, see the examples below:

Situation	Tom's Actions	Claire's Actions
Assessment	Usually gets information from old notes and families. He never asks the persons about their own health or nursing-care needs.	Explains assessment, provides written information, and asks persons with dementia for their consent to proceed where she can.
Being safe in bed	Risk assessment always scores as high risk so he fits bed rails and ensures they are up.	Risk assessment is used as a guide along with assessment of knowing what is used at home.
Walking and/or wandering around	Generally accompanies persons back to a communal area or their bed area if he sees them walking around or wandering, especially if they are going towards reception or doors.	Sees providing a safe space as important in promotion of walking and wandering.
Personal hygiene	Tells the person they are having personal care when he feels it is the right time.	Negotiates with the person to see what they would like to do. Will generally accept if someone declines personal care and return at a later time to offer it again.
Reports, discharge planning or multi-disciplinary team discussions	Uses language and selects examples that portrays the persons as a high risk and as 'hard work'. Tends to focus on what persons cannot do and the problems they cause staff and others.	Uses language that is respectful and conveys person's dignity. Tends to focus on what persons can do and how they try to problem-solve for themselves.
Supervising students	Offers a negative picture of nursing older people, where it is about crisis management and the nurses being constantly on their guard against what the persons might be doing wrong or that might cause them harm. Role models poor appreciation of how persons dementia experience the world and does not invest in dementia-sensitive processes.	Offers a more positive picture of nursing older people based on helping older people to achieve what they want and to remain independent in whatever ways are important to them. Emphasises an appreciation how persons with dementia experience the world, the processes of communication and negotiation.

All persons bring with them, into their preparation to become a registered nurse, sets of beliefs and values about many things, some of which they will be aware of and some they will not. Many values stem from childhood and experiences of parenting/carers. You might like to consider your own parents or significant carers in your childhood; the values they have/had; and how this has influenced your values and beliefs at this stage in your life and work. It is also possible to ask nurses you work with if they will talk with you about their values and how they feature in their day-to-day work. You can also observe nurses and other health and social care professionals at work (also carers and volunteers) to see if their values shine through. Those who have reflected and clarified their values will generally offer you more articulate descriptions. Both Tom and Claire's actions are certainly consistent with their values, but they are both practising in different ways, using different processes and will achieve different outcomes because of their values base.

Clarifying your values

Clarifying values and beliefs about nursing older people with mental health needs is vital for several reasons. First, as I have already suggested, it is necessary to establish what values and beliefs you bring with you into nursing, ensuring that decisions and actions are value-based and to identify which ones you could be exploring in order to develop a less-biased or more balanced position. Some values and beliefs might also be linked to fears. So, a fear associated with, for example, people defecating or with physical aggression will need to be explored and worked on. Otherwise, you might find yourself avoiding those situations or engaging with patients in a non-authentic and non-therapeutic way.

Being clear about what you value and believe about nursing can hold you in good stead in practice where you might see care given by members of the health-care team (including registered nurses) that is different to that which you have been learning about. Developing critical insight into what constitutes good practice and unsatisfactory practice is an essential skill in nursing, as this helps to set personal standards to work along with professionally required standards laid down to nurses by the Nursing and Midwifery Council. Some research shows that nurses who are clear about their values and beliefs, and who put these into action in their day-to-day work with older people are more committed to their work and to their patients (McCance, 1997). What we see, hear, read, experience, and reflect upon interacts with our beliefs about something. This belief gives us an understanding or misunderstanding which, in turn, allows us to appraise its worth (or value). The value we place on something is not always correct due to a variety of influences such as mis-understanding, lack of experience, miscommunication and being misled by another person's values and beliefs. Ghaye (2005, p. 132) suggests that there are six potential concerns associated with values. Some practitioners and teams can be blind to their values, whilst others can have so many values there is values confusion, then others make only token gestures to putting values in the centre of their practice, and values can also be abused to achieve conflict or conquests over the values of others which can mean some feel a sense of alienation in respect to their own values.

Ageism

A central value, to be examined when choosing to work with older people, is ageism. Ageism is pervasive in western cultures and affects all age groups but is most profound in older people (Heath, 1999, p. 12). Ageism, often referred to as age discrimination, exists in many areas of life such as consumerism, design, crime, media, civic and voluntary life and politics. It is an abuse of human rights and causes personal suffering and hardship and cultural and economic problems. A recent survey by Age Concern (2005) found that:

- Twenty-nine per cent of people reported suffering age discrimination as opposed to any other form of discrimination.
- After the age of 55, people were nearly twice as likely to have experienced age prejudice than any other form of discrimination.
- Nearly 30% of people believed that there is more prejudice against the old than 5 years ago.
- People believed that age discrimination will continue to get worse.
- One-third of people thought that the demographic shift towards an older society would make life worse in terms of standards of living, security, health, jobs and education
- One in three respondents said they viewed the over 70s as incompetent and incapable.

A new law came into effect on 1 October 2006. The Employment Equality (Age) Regulations (2006) came into force in England, Wales and Scotland. Although, the regulations will provide protection against age discrimination in employment, training and adult education, for people of all ages, it does not affect health care.

As a professional it is important that you can describe your values and beliefs clearly and concisely. Knowing your values and beliefs can be useful in practice, for academic work and in a range of other situations (see next section), so it is worthwhile spending some time investing in a method to achieve clarification. A values clarification exercise (Warfield and Manley, 1990; Manley, 1992) is a tool frequently used within practice development for developing a common shared vision and purpose. It can be used for developing a common vision about many different areas (see Dewing et al., 2006). However, the same tool can also be used by individual nurses and student nurses to clarify their own values and beliefs. A values clarification exercise can provide the starting-point for personal change in the workplace, as our values and beliefs influence our behaviour. Though making explicit our values and beliefs, we are taking the first steps to making them a reality in our work with patients and more generally in our practice in the workplace. A match between what we say we believe and what we do is one of the hallmarks of effective individuals, teams and organisations (Manley, 2000). A simple tool can enable nurses to undertake their own values clarification as a way of clarifying their personal vision of nursing.

What does a values clarification exercise look like?

This always starts with a stem to help identify the main/ultimate purpose, for example 'I/we believe the ultimate purpose of nursing older people with mental health needs is …' This stem would always be followed by a second stem which identifies how the purpose can be achieved, for example 'I/we believe this purpose can be achieved by …' A number of other stems would usually be included depending on the purpose of the exercise (see Table 4.2 for the complete tool adapted for this context). What you end up with is a set of categories that you shape into a summary statement of your values, as shown in the following example.

Table 4.2 Values and beliefs tool

> - I believe the ultimate purpose of nursing older people with mental-health needs is:
> - I believe this purpose is best achieved by:
> - I believe my contribution to this purpose is:
> - I believe that to enhance my contribution, I need to:
>
> *Method*
> If you are doing this exercise for yourself, allow about 30–60 min and find a quiet or creative space where you can think and make notes. Take a separate piece of paper for each of the four stems given above and write the stem at the top of each sheet (one stem per sheet). Under each of the stems, make notes of your responses to each one. Keep each response as a separate sentence or bullet point.
>   Look again at what you have written and organise your sentences and responses into similar or alike categories. Give each category a title or name that represents as far as possible all the responses. You might end up with a number of categories and titles on each sheet of paper.
>   Look again at the categories and see if there is any priority to them. Does one seem more important than another? Do you want to change any of the terms? You could discuss your categories with a friend or mentor to help you reflect further.
>   Write a draft summary statement of your values and beliefs using the stems given above.
>   Review the draft statement and edit it until it is clear and concise but captures your values and beliefs.
>   Note: where the activity is used in a group, a similar process is used. The emergent statement may inform the way a team organises itself and its work or be used as a framework to critique practice of a team to establish variance between discussed values and those actually experienced. More broadly, it can be used as a framework for curriculum or research work or to inform the direction and priorities of systematic practice development.

Values and evidence base

Nurses need to look at the relationship between their values and beliefs and knowledge, no matter how experienced they are. For example, I had thought

Example

Categories:

I believe the ultimate purpose of nursing older people with mental-health needs is: assessment, quality service, well-trained staff, person-centred care and needs-led service. I believe this purpose is best achieved by: team work, person-centredness, supportive management, leadership, development, and education.

I believe my contribution to this purpose is: gain knowledge to work as a competent registered nurse, be open to new experiences and learning. I believe that to enhance my contribution I need to: be a life-long learner, build up an evidence base, involve patients and develop reflective practice.

Summary draft statement:

I believe the ultimate purpose of nursing older people with mental-health needs is to provide a needs-led and person-centred service, beginning with quality assessment that is delivered by well-prepared staff. This is best achieved by person-centred teams with well-prepared and continuously developing staff who have clear leadership and a supportive management.

My contribution to this purpose is to gain knowledge and skills to work as a competent registered nurse, and be open to learning. I recognise that I will need to commit to be a life–long learner and build up an evidence base for my practice and that I will need to involve and learn from patients and develop reflective practice.

(Note the small improvements in some of the terms used between the category statements and the summary draft statement)

I was clear about what my values and beliefs were on what person-centred nursing was. However, quite recently, during the course of doing a literature review on the concepts of person and personhood, I became more aware that my knowledge was limited, and new knowledge I was acquiring was challenging some of my existing values and beliefs. This caused me to reflect deeply on my values and beliefs. The outcome, on this occasion, was that I adapted in some way my beliefs about what a person is and clarified my values on personhood and what this means for me as a person-centred practitioner and practice-developer. Thus, if I state I believe I am a person-centred practitioner, as a professional I am obliged to look at my beliefs to see if they are congruent with what is already known about the area. Reflecting on values and beliefs is vital but it must also be as part of a dialogue with other sources of evidence.

Having values and working with them

Knowing what your values are is not the end-point for a nurse – just the starting-point for a life-long relationship. There can easily be or gradually develop over time, a gap or dissonance between what we say we value and how much we act according to what we say we value. Constantly acting in ways that emphasise the gap between these two can result in stress is a negative means of coping, and results in a lack of authenticity as a person and a nurse. Lack of authenticity often stems from a lack of awareness in the values or beliefs at the core of 'who I am'. Additionally, when we are not centered in who we are and what we believe and value, challenge and change are often a threat. Future practitioners and leaders in nursing cannot afford to feel overly threatened by challenge, feel unable to make personal transitions and transformations or not adapt to new evidence supporting best practice.

An effective nursing leader provides spirit and meaning to others through reinforcing shared values and challenging values that are not consistent with the team's shared values for practice. When our values are not in focus, our energy can become easily dispersed, making it tougher to motivate and mobilise ourselves, never mind anyone else. Core values provide a context for continuous growth and development that takes us toward our vision. Our core values project forward to become our vision for how we would like things to be. Developing and communicating a vision is a behaviour associated with transformational leadership (Manley, 1997). Knowing what our values and beliefs are is only the beginning of processes of positive change. Putting values and beliefs into practice involves overcoming a number of barriers which exist in both ourselves and our workplaces. Nurses who can effectively dismantling barriers and recognise the gaps or dissonance between what their teams say they believe, what they say they do, and what they actually do are worth learning from. This characteristic of values-based action is central to emancipatory practice development, an approach to practice development based on critical social science and one which claims to achieve sustainable change in the workplace (Manley and McCormack, 2003).

From values to action

The history of nursing older people with mental health needs has been associated with what are now regarded as negative values and beliefs about older people (Nolan 2003, p. 5). Kitwood concludes, historical patterns in care of older people with mental health needs in western cultures means that all care practice still has attributes of moral deficit, warehousing and unnecessary use of the medical model. Although somewhat a generalisation, the way we care for older people, especially those with mental health needs, still needs attention both at the practitioner–patient interface and more widely at a policy interface (Bosanquet, 2001; Harriot, 2006). Mental Health Nursing must move away from traditional models of care and working practices to a more positive values-based approach.

The Chief Nursing Officers Review of Mental Health Nursing (Department of Health 2006) called *From Values to Action* is underpinned by the idea that values of Mental Health Nursing need to be re-visioned and that the 'new' values need to inform every aspect of practice (p. 11). Further, patient-centredness is said to be core to this new set of values (p. 16). The review calls on Mental Health Nurses to reflect on their values in these key areas:

- the Recovery Approach to practice;
- partnership working with users (valuing aims of the user and offering meaningful choices);
- social inclusion (particularly tackling social stigma);
- being optimistic about the possibility for recovery.

It should be noted that recovery is not the recovery in terms of cure from disease or illness but more of a psychosocial, spiritual recovery – regaining a sense of wholeness or completeness.

Currently, the beliefs around user- or person-centredness are a popular underpinning for practice. Describing what constitutes person-centred values is not always as easy as it seems, and confusion with values makes translation into practice more challenging (see Case Study 4.3).

Values enabling person-centredness

The basis for person-centred care is said to be nurturing personhood (Dewing 2004; McCormack, 2004). Kitwood's definition of personhood is: 'a position or social relationship that is bestowed on one human being by "others", in the context of relationship and social being' Kitwood (1997, p. 8).

Kitwood's definition of personhood suggests that being a person is both a status to which human beings aspire and a process. You can feel you have status as a person (the social being) but that status is fundamentally affected by the processes others use that either adds to or takes way from your identity as a person. Thus, the core of person-centredness is twofold: first, the attributes we regard as essential for a human to be regarded as being worthy of inclusion as a social being; second, the sort of relationships we have. As Kitwood (1997) argued, older human beings/persons with dementia and other mental health disabilities push our society to the limit in terms of what it is prepared to accept in regard to personhood status. In the example with Tom and Claire, Tom is probably not person-centred, at least when it comes to older people with dementia, whereas Claire probably is, at least in the situations shown above.

Knowing what our values are and having person-centred values can enable nurses to act in the best interests of older people, especially in complex situations where there are multiple factors and agendas at play. Asking yourself 'In this situation, what are the core values by which I/we need to make a decision and act on?' can form a guide. Asking others the same question can also help in group or team discussions. To be truly person-centred, the question can be rephrased as 'In this situation, what are the core values of *the older person* on which I/we need to make a decision and act on?' However, even then, where others who may have different values are also involved, decision-making can still be problematic. But what is important is that the processes and underpinning values have been openly addressed. Consider how this next scenario might challenge certain values and beliefs about older persons and require nurses to be clear about their values and beliefs.

Case study 4.3

Mrs O, a widow for 20 years, aged 82, has a probable dementia of the Alzheimer's type. She lives in a care home and her family have little contact with her. She has had an on–off very intimate and satisfying relationship with a male resident for the last two years. About 4 months ago, he called off the relationship, as he felt she was making too many sexual demands on him. Mrs O now regularly makes approaches to several male residents where she masturbates herself and attempts to do the same to the men. The home has a philosophy that stresses person-centredness and enabling older people to have fulfilling relationships and to live a fulfilling life.

Many staff find Mrs O's behaviour difficult and are embarrassed when they encounter it. Mrs O has become the regular topic of conversation at handovers and at the staff-support group. Staff know that other residents are discussing her behaviour. Staff have, without realising it, withdrawn from Mrs O. She gets minimal staff time and little demonstration of affection, warmth or value as a person. There are now demands from staff that she is 'put on' medication to stop her inappropriate behaviour.

Conclusions

Core values concerned with mental health and older people's nursing are accepted as inherently good, for example, dignity choice, independence and autonomy. However, they become extremely complex in their translation to practice (Nolan et al., 2001, p. 11) and as shown in this chapter. Nurses who know and attend to clarifying their values, ensure their actions are values-based and are authentic and consistent in the way they practise, but still might not be offering person-centred or evidence-based care. Nurses who have person-centred values and reflect on their values against evidence, will work to ensure they ground their nursing care in working with the beliefs and values of older people as far as they can and offer evidence-based care – or so I believe! Nurses must ensure that they work collaboratively as part of a team and establish shared values and beliefs so that the team's approach and the older person's experience of care are consistent.

Resources

http://www.ageconcern.org.uk/AgeConcern/ageism.asp highlights forms of ageism in the UK and what can be done about it.
http://www.mentalhealth.org.uk/exists to help people survive, recover from and prevent mental health problems.
http://www.dh.gov.uk/PolicyAndGuidance/HealthAndSocialCareTopics/Older PeoplesServices/OlderPeopleArticle/fs/en?CONTENT_ID=4002284andchk=q4tpUL Standard Seven: Mental Health and Older People.

http://www.annalsoflongtermcare.com/article/4786 contains a checklist for cultural sensitive care with older people living in care homes

References

Age Concern. (2005) *How Ageist is Britain?* London, Age Concern.

Andrews, M. M. and Herberg, P. (1999) Transcultural nursing care. In: *Transcultural Concepts in Nursing Care*, 3rd edn (A. Andrews and J.S. Boyle, eds). Philadelphia, PA, Lippincott, pp. 25–27.

Bosanquet, N. (2001) The socioeconomic impact of Alzheimer's disease. *International Journal of Geriatric Psychiatry* **16**, 249–253.

Department of Health (2006) *From Values to Action: The Chief Nursing Officer's Review of Mental Health Nursing*. London, Department of Health.

Dewing, J. (2004) Concerns relating to the application of frameworks to promote person-centredness in nursing with older people. *Journal of Clinical Nursing* **13** (*International Journal of Older Peoples Nursing* s1), 39–44.

Dewing, J., Brooks, J. and Riddaway, I. (2006) Involving older people in practice development. Practice: An Evaluation of an Intermediate Care Service and its Multi- disciplinary Practice. *Practice Development in Health Care Journal* **5** (3), 156–174.

Ghaye, T. (2005) *Developing the Reflective Healthcare Team*. Oxford. Blackwell.

Harriot, H. H. (2006) Old age, successful ageing and the problem of significance. *Journal of the European Ethics Network* **13** (1), 119–143.

Heath, H. (1999) Perspectives on ageing and older people In: *Healthy Ageing: Nursing Older People* (H. Heath and I. Schofield, eds). London, Mosby, pp. 3–20.

Higgs, J. and Andresen, L. (2001) The knower, the knowing and the known: threads in the woven tapestry of knowledge. In: *Practice Knowledge and Expertise in the Health Professions* (J. Higgs and A. Titchen, eds). London, Butterworth-Heinemann.

Kitwood, T. (1997) *Dementia Reconsidered: the Person Comes First*. Buckingham, UK, Open University Press.

Ludwick, R. and Cipriano-Silva, M. (2000) Nursing around the world: Cultural values and ethical conflicts. *Journal of Issues in Nursing*, 14 August. http://www.nursingworld. org/ojin/ethicol/ethics_4.htm

McCance, T. (1997) Caring: dealing with a difficult concept. *International Journal of Nursing Studies* **34** (4), 241–248.

McCormack, B. (2004) Person-centredness in gerontological nursing: an overview of the literature. *Journal of Clinical Nursing* **13** (*International Journal of Older Peoples Nursing* s1), 31–38

McCormack, B. (2005) Underpinning values. In: *Older People: Assessment for Health Care and Social Care* (H. Heath and R. Watson, eds). London, Age Concern, pp. 44–53.

Manley, K. (1992) Quality assurance: the pathway to excellence in nursing In: *Nursing Care The Challenge to Change* (eds. G. Brykczinska and M. Jolley) London, Edward Arnold.

Manley, K. (1997) A conceptual framework for advanced practice: an action research project operationalising an advanced practitioner/consultant nurse role. *Journal of Clinical Nursing* **6** (2), 179–190.

Manley, K. and McCormack, B. (2003) Practice development: Purpose, Methodology, Facilitation and Evaluation Nursing in critical care **8** (1), 22–29.

Manley, K. (2000) *Organisational Culture and Consultant Nurse Outcomes: Part 1 Organisational Culture*. London, RCN.

Nolan, M., Davis, S. and Grant, G. (2001) Quality of care, quality of life. In: *Working with Older People and Their Families* (M. Nolan, S. Davis and G. Grant, eds). Buckingham, UK, Open University Press, pp. 4–18.

Nolan, P. (2003) Voices form the past. In: *Community Mental Health Nursing and Dementia Care* (J. Keady, C. Clarke and T. Adams, eds). Maidenhead, UK, Open University Press, pp. 3–16.

Warfield, C. and Manley, K. (1990) Developing a new philosophy in the NDU. *Nursing Standard* **4** (41), 27–30.

Chapter 5
Approaches to Help, Support and Care

Elizabeth Collier

Introduction

What is support? What is care? Words that are quick and easy to speak, words that textbooks tell us we should provide, words that we write in care plans, in clinical correspondence, philosophies, operational statements and assignments. But what do support and care mean? In our personal lives, we offer support to our friends and relatives. Sometimes in times of extreme stress, we want to offer support but feel completely impotent. The best support we can offer may be a letter or card, a token of recognition, an occasional phone call letting the person know we are there and available; sometimes it may be being able to recognise when to leave some space – that we are not the best persons to provide help. A student recently wrote in an assignment reflection that she had spent much time sitting with a client in her room in silence and felt this impotence. She was very surprised but gratified to find out much later from the client that she had really helped her by sitting with her in silence. This chapter attempts to focus on such fundamental skills. It attempts to maintain a connection with the meaning of help, support and care; things that are often intended but we have failed to provide, evidenced by the stories of the experiences of older adults. To strive to provide true support and care, we require continuing development of our self-awareness, to understand that it is the little things that count (Macleod, 1994). Hope, support and information have been found to be the most helpful to recovery, and ignorance and stigma the greatest hindrance (Coyne Plum, 1987). Our best approach therefore may be to be continually open and willing to recognise and challenge our own ignorance and contributions to stigmatising people.

We should be constantly willing to consider that we are prejudiced and discriminatory, even when we believe we are not. The document 'Turning your back on us' (Gilchrist, 1999) shows us how health professionals do practise in a discriminatory way through the distressing stories of patients and relatives. The staff that are referred to are unlikely to be purposefully cruel and arguably mortified, if they thought they had caused such distress. But good intentions are not good enough. We should explore our attitudes and behaviour again and again.

This chapter focuses on people first, rather than theory, using people's names as subheadings, as the people shape any approaches to support and care. As a carer recently indicated to me, 'Sometimes, it's enough just to listen and let them [carers] offload; other times they may need some practical help or advice. The skill is to know the difference.' This chapter draws on both clinical and teaching experience.

Think about Mrs Gordon.

Mrs Jane Gordon

Mrs Gordon has been married since she was aged 18 and she is now 75. She has been feeling confused lately, as she is unhappy in her relationship. She is uncomfortable about some aspects of her sexual relationship, plus she feels that her husband has always been a bully and has undermined her all their married life. In addition, she thinks that some of her confusion arises out of her own questions about her sexuality that she has avoided all her life. Her refusal to have sex has led to arguments with her partner, and she thinks that maybe they should end the marriage. Her confusion and distress are too great for her to bear.

Before this is discussed, consider your responses to the following questions:

- What is your instinctive reaction to this scenario?
- What advice would you give Jane if she asked you?
- Is this the same advice you would give to a 30-year-old who has been married since she was 18?
- Is the advice you would give Jane based on (a) your own values or (b) Jane's expressed needs?

Table 5.1 shows a summary of responses to this scenario that has been collected in a classroom situation. It represents the responses of approximately 60 student mental health nurses who completed the same scenario with people of different ages, i.e. Jane as a 16-, 30- and 75-year-old (groups did not know that their Jane was a different age than the next group). The discussion that followed considered why such different advice would be considered given the reported problem. It can be seen that for people of different ages, there are similarities and differences. We may modify our interactions based on the dynamics of the relationship, e.g. if the person is perceived as much younger or much older than ourselves. This is understandable and acceptable, but not the issue. The issue is: is it alright to use a different set of rules to make decisions about the help we provide based only on (real or perceived) chronological age? There are many influences at work. One example is of the interpretation of the word 'confusion'. For the 16- and 30-year-old Jane, this was interpreted as a general indication of being unsure; for Jane, the 75-year-old, this was interpreted in the context of 'dementia', a symptom of something else. Why? There is nothing in this scenario that suggests any pathological problems at all. Interestingly, the

Table 5.1 Summary of responses to a scenario regarding people of different ages

16-year-old girl	30-year-old woman	75-year-old woman
Confusion due to hormones	Why does she think he is a bully?	Why is she confused?
Refer to Child and Adolescent Mental Health Services	Other relationships have been different, or is it her issue/assess mood and confusion?	Psychiatric or neurological assessment
Psychological abuse/peer pressure/right to say no	Advocacy, assertiveness training	Not surprised about her feelings given bullying
Talk about sexual orientation	Exploration of self and sexuality	Sex drive gone, so not an issue
Discuss contraception; give information, e.g. Brook advisory centre, puberty	Learn about self; sort sexual feelings out	Sexual desire misplaced from need for friendship
Involve parents	Peer and family involvement/women's support group	Advise her to discuss with husband/social outlet, e.g. bingo, ballroom dancing
Too young to know what she wants/do what she feels/talk about sexual orientation	Break/end the relationship	Relationship not to end; been married too long and financially dependent
Get counselling	Counselling (relate) and one-to-one counselling	Counselling and support

youngest and the oldest were more likely to be referred to specialist mental health services, but it was consistent that the 75-year-old Jane was considered to need neurological or psychiatric assessment. Sometimes her sexuality was disregarded altogether and reinterpreted as *her* misinterpretation for friendship. Some were confused by the exercise as '75-year-olds don't have sex, and it's not realistic', despite evidence such as Beckman et al. (2005) where it was found that 95% ($n = 563$) of people over 70 years of age continue to have sexual needs and interests, and also Walker et al. (2005) who found that 20% of their sample (30 questionnaires returned) had had intercourse within the past month, and 40% had masturbated (half men, half women). Although there was one occasion when the issue for trial separation was identified for the 75-year-old, it can be seen that the general responses are different. Why is it so difficult to listen and understand, instead of reinterpreting reality in our own world view? Clearly, for someone who is distressed and asks for help in such a situation, they need to be taken seriously, be able to discuss their feelings in detail and be supported to reach any decisions that make the most sense to them. So, how can people like Jane be supported and cared for?

One potential problem here is that reactions to this scenario can be emotional and based on personal value systems rather than objective and practical, as we would expect in a professional context. This illustrates potential problems in

Box 5.1   Reflective exercise

- Does it cause me any anxiety to let older people make their own decisions?
- Do I talk differently in any way to older people than to people similar to myself in age?
- Do I modify the information, advice and interventions I provide older people?
- What are my personal influences/experience that influence how I interact with older people?
- What language do I use in my personal life relating to older people, and how does this influence my professional life?
- Does my practice area cite age restrictions in any policies?
- Can I objectively justify these responses?

providing support and care to someone in Jane's position and essentially is an example of indirect age discrimination; to help Jane, this discriminatory attitude has to be acknowledged and learned from. To think through your own responses, complete the reflective exercise in Box 5.1.

The principles of age discrimination highlighted in this scenario and Table 5.1 apply to all the following scenarios, but are potentially compounded by any other discrimination that can occur on the grounds of mental illness, ethnicity, disability or sexuality.

Mr Raj Josephs

Mr Josephs' wife Elizabeth has been diagnosed with Alzheimer's disease for some time. They live in their own home and have help from mental health services. Every 8 weeks, Mrs Josephs spends a week in respite care in a nursing home.

Situations such as that of Mr Josephs are very common. In such a case, nurses have the mental-heath needs of at least two people to consider and address. As a friend or relative, such a situation can leave people feeling guilty and hopeless. A carer's perspective and their mental health needs are not always very well considered, despite the abundance of literature acknowledging their needs, but in practice it may be that the true cost to them is not understood. There is a risk by practitioners to consider the 'burden' of caring. Of course, there are people who may very well describe this as a burden and may need help to decide what they will do, but for many people this situation represents a developmental stage of a relationship, finding new things out about each other and finding new ways to live together. It may be unsupportive to try to persuade someone they need a rest, to suggest they separate from their partner, when this is not a solution that meets their needs. The carer knows what is best within the relationship they have, far better than any visiting practitioner. Good intentions or best-interest arguments from a professional perspective are not necessarily helpful to the carer.

What does help? It is often persuasive as practitioners to think of sophisticated therapies, when in fact such situations call for very practical approaches to mental health promotion for the carer and client. As the paper 'It's the little things that count' emphasises (Macleod, 1994), attention to detail in everyday life is the most

Table 5.2 Responses given by carers about things that help the least/most

Things that help the most	Things that do not help/caused difficulties
Finding out we could use disabled toilets if we went out	Hiding behind 'confidentiality' as an excuse not to provide information
Services of a CPN team after diagnosis	Do not provide any false hope; do not suggest things early on that may not actually be achievable (maybe because of funding issues) – unfulfilled promises
First-class continuing care; no smells at the home; no bed sores; good nutrition	Expectations that were not met, e.g. nurse not getting back to me with information as she had said she would
Family support	Periodic assessment appointments not being honoured and feeling they were only for staff's benefit, not ours
Admiral nurses	
Understand and accept some selfishness without judgement – self preservation	
Give direct honest answers; if you don't know, say so	
Knowing what services are available and how to access them	
Alzheimer's Society support group; not being alone and feeling someone actually cares	

productive and helpful approach to care. At an Alzheimer's Society carer-support group recently, a group of carers were asked 'What helps/helped the most?' and 'What helps/helped the least? The responses can be seen in Table 5.2.

As a privileged observer to this group, it was a salutary reminder of the reality of the hidden pain that thousands of people who have to care for a relative at home with a dementia are going through on an hourly basis everyday. There appeared to be anger, resignation, upset and tears, bitterness, brutal honesty, love and frustration. It was clear that any burden that was felt was a burden not so much of caring, but of guilt. What was also clear was that help had to be very much related to understanding the actual relationship of the people involved. There seemed to be a story about how people had to learn to communicate again, a lesson that professionals should listen to, an acceptance that the person with dementia was changing against everyone's will, you could not change them, so the only person who could change to make things better was you, the family member/carer and that you have to adapt to life now and its limitations. As a professional involved, it is sometimes difficult to see past one's own stresses of the 'job' to the reason for the job in the first place. The default position when helping carers and their relatives has to be to believe the carer absolutely. There was frustration in relation to the disregard of the carer's account, where medical staff often relied on high scores on mini-mental-state examinations for example to inform their opinions, rather than the descriptions from carers that such apparent presence of mind would most definitely not be the picture later in the day, People made creative inroads into managing their situations to try to improve them for everyone. For example, one person talked of finding the 'magic word', the particular suggestion, phrase or word that would have a calming or distracting effect. This seemed to be recognised by other people who agreed that this does take time, and you have to try many different things (personal to you and the relative) to discover it. For one person, this was saying, 'come on let's put the kettle on, and I'll make you a nice cup of tea', a technique that resulted on one occasion from his relative stopping screaming and screaming on the path at the front of their house. Other techniques were very personal and could only be effective between the people involved in the context of their relationship. This has to be respected and accepted. Professional staff may feel some conflict with their professional values or responsibilities to the 'patient', the person diagnosed with dementia but, following these feelings, may only be unsupportive to the carer. One example of this is the issue of confidentiality. As can be seen in Table 5.2, 'hiding behind confidentiality as an excuse not to provide information' is one of the issues that has been identified as being the most unhelpful. Weighing up the issues and an honest conversation about this with both people involved is perhaps the most helpful approach. The NHS code of practice on confidentiality (Department of Health, 2003) actually states:

'If a patient is unable to give consent or communicate a decision … due to mental condition …, the health professionals concerned must make a decision about the use of the information. This needs to take into account the patient's best interests … be informed by the views of the carers.' (Annex B, pp. 26 and 31)

In addition to the questions in Table 5.2, carers were also asked: what [student] nurses should know about carers experience, what was the worse thing they could do and what was the best thing they could do to help. Table 5.3 shows the responses.

Thinking of the best way to help in the context of a personal relationship is most important, whether these relationships are daughter–mother or husband–wife; Box 5.2 shows some examples of approaches that can be used. To help people, assumptions should not be made or blanket approaches used; any interventions suggested to help need to be in keeping with their shared values.

In addition, the Alzheimer's Society Newsletter (2005) published a carer's list of eight care-giving maxims for dealing with perplexing behaviour. Clearly, the attention to the carer will have an effect for the quality of the life of the person with dementia. The suggestions made by a carer were:

- Don't try to stop people with dementia doing something just because it isn't being done 'properly'. Don't take over; give them time to do things in their own way and at their own pace.
- People with dementia understand far more than they are ever given credit for. Take care what is said in their presence and don't exclude them from conversations or decisions.

- It is very easy to confuse 'caring' with 'controlling' – we all hate the sense that someone is controlling our lives. If someone cannot find the words to protest, then resistance or aggressive action will ensue.
- Ask the question 'Who is it a problem for: us or them?' If the answer is us, then we should be able to let things ride and not argue to contradict (does it really matter that someone eats mashed potato with their fingers or wants to go to bed with their trousers on?).
- Preserve autonomy for as long as possible by giving choices, e.g. what clothes to wear. Celebrate what the person can still do, rather than bemoan what they can't (is the bottle half full or half empty?).
- There is nearly always a reason for agitation, often something or somebody in the environment. Try to spot the cause and change it if possible. If you encounter resistance, walk away and try again later.
- If the person with dementia cannot enter our world, we must enter theirs and affirm it. Forget reality orientation – what day it is, who the prime minister is, who cares? Be prepared to time-travel backwards into their personal history and their 'real' world. Indulge in a few white lies if necessary. When was it a sin to make someone happy?
- Look behind the illness and reach out to the frightened person still in there who needs to feel secure, respected and cherished.

Professionals can be easily distracted by anxiety around legal and ethical responsibilities. This can be a source of anger, frustration and stress for a carer who needs information. A compromise must be reached with the carer in regard to a mutual understanding of each other's constraints and duties. A carer's perspective in a situation such as this is often the best evidence for professional approach to care, as illustrated in the carer's view above.

Table 5. 3 Responses given by carers about nurses

Nurses should know	Best thing they can do	Worst thing they can do
Do not make assumptions about the help people need; everyone is different. Listen to carers	Walk in carers' shoes: practical experience is worth a thousand text books Get a placement with admiral nurse or CPN	Talking to the carer as if the person they are caring for is not there Believe that attending lectures or extensive reading will teach them what is necessary
Know about carers' emotional experience	Attend a carers' group	Pretend it does not exist
Know about carers' practical problems	Ask the Alzheimer's Society if you can meet at least one carer	
Know what Alzheimer's disease is and how it may end eventually		

Box 5.2   Examples of approaches

- James's wife would not get out of bed. A routine was planned and expectations created. Weekends were for staying-in-bed time, and week days were for doing things – he would keep a calendar on the bedroom wall, and instead of asking her if she wanted to get up, he would say, 'Oh it's Tuesday today; it's our go-to-the-library day; I'll get your clothes, and we can get ready'. On Saturdays he would again state what would happen, 'It's Saturday, lay-in day; I'll call you when lunch is ready'.
- Mary kept phoning her daughter literally every 10 min, not remembering the conversation 5 min previously and starting the same conversation again. Her daughter could not cope with this, as it was very stressful and distressing. She used an answer machine to take the calls and called her mother just once a day in the evening. Her mother was not distressed, as she did not remember that she had called 60 times previously.
- Howard's wife lives in a nursing home. He spends a lot of time with her each day. When he goes on holiday with his son, he leaves a tape recorder that the staff play to his wife each morning, where he says 'Come on Helen; get up; it's breakfast time' and at night he reads a prayer to her when she goes to bed.

Mrs Rose Smith

Mrs Rose Smith is a retired teacher. She moved to the UK from Jamaica only recently to be near to her daughter after her husband died age 79. She has been living alone in a flat and spending her time helping with various community projects at her local church. She has recently come to the attention of the mental health service after a referral from her GP indicating that she believes she is in contact with her sister who has been dead for 15 years. Her preoccupation with this has become so great that it has led to neglect of her usual personal standards of being well dressed, hair done and looking generally smart, as well as not cooking and not eating well. She has lost a large amount of weight. She is attending a day hospital at present for a mental health assessment. To help Mrs Smith, the cultural context of her experiences must be understood. If an effort is not made to understand this, then she cannot be supported or helped. As a professional, we are most usually expected to complete certain quite structured assessments. This can easily distract us from any focus on mental health promotion, when in fact this may be the most effective approach to helping a person and achieving the aim of supporting them to live at home successfully. Consider Mrs Smith from a mental health promotion point of view, rather than a mental health assessment point of view.

List your thoughts in relation to the question:

- What are the potential risks to Mrs Smith's mental health and happiness?
- Do you think your responses are/would be the same as those Mrs Smith would describe?
- Imagine you are Mrs Smith.
- What are the risks to your health and happiness? List your thoughts.
  How do your two lists of responses compare?
  As a professional your responses may include issues such as:
- isolation; feeling lost and lonely;
- lack of culturally sensitive social networks;

- bereavement; loss of and feelings for;
  - long-term home;
  - husband;
  - sister;
  - familiar culture, place, sights, sounds and smells;
- reduced self-esteem.

In considering how Mrs Smith may see things, the following could help minimise these risks:

- Learn to understand her perspective on what is happening to her and her explanations of her feelings about her situation.
- Accompany her to the hairdresser (a specialist in Afro-Caribbean hair).
- Accompany her to do her washing and ironing.
- Find out feelings towards her involvement with the church – if they are positive, ensure contact is maintained.
- Find out support that the daughter can offer.
- Check out cultural links and support available in her area and put her in touch, e.g. African Caribbean centres.
- Intellectual needs; access to Jamaican or Christian literature (depending on her preference).
- Access to Jamaican or Christian music.
- Talk with her about her relationship with her sister.
- What does she want for her future? Identify possible resources that could contribute to achieving this.

In addition to the above, describe *how* you will go about achieving this, e.g. how will you learn to understand her perspective on what is happening to her and her feelings about her situation? How will you ensure she has access to a choice of literature and music that includes that of Jamaican or Christian origin. List the actions that you would take to achieve this.

This kind of attention to detail and illustration of your thoughtfulness could make all the difference to Mrs Smith and her family. The affect of such behaviours is not necessarily quantifiable, but their absence may create the atmosphere within which a useful helping relationship is developed or not; a feeling about whether someone feels cared for or not. Even if the help is not successful in terms of health outcomes, i.e. Mrs Smith's symptoms appear unchanged, its impact can remain influential in the experience of care that she and her family feel they are getting and have an effect on long-term satisfaction and engagement.

It would not be entirely surprising if Mrs Smith found herself with a medical diagnosis of clinical depression or psychosis and was prescribed medication. The medical model is very powerful and shapes our health services. It can, however, potentially conflict with the intention to help. How can Mrs Smith be helped? Her cultural values may include a belief in telepathy and a relationship with relatives who have died. An understanding of this thorough dialogue will be most helpful (the opposite of most unhelpful to her, that is, relying on an understanding of her 'symptoms' that summarise her experiences as a delusion).

The professional should be open to an education about Mrs Smith's cultural and personal values. Clearly, her behaviour in the scenario has brought her to the attention of health-care services. An understanding of how she interprets what is happening to her is the key to mental well-being, as she may not see it as a mental health issue at all. The day hospital may be an alien and isolating experience for her where opportunities for mixing with people from similar cultural backgrounds are absent, perhaps unlike her experiences at church. The term 'mental health' may be completely alien, as it is for many people. Terms of mental health or ill health have been shown to be disregarded or completely unknown for some black Afro-Caribbean people. Marwaha and Livingstone (2002) interviewed 40 white British and black Afro-Caribbean people, half of whom had been depressed, using vignettes describing an older man with depression and a woman with psychosis. Findings suggested that most of the black Afro-Caribbean people did not consider depression an illness; nor did they think psychiatric services were appropriate, as they thought mental health services were for dealing with violent people and that spiritual help would be more appropriate.

Our mental health world is very familiar to us, and we easily forget that it is a completely frightening alien world for most of the people we come into contact with who do not understand the language or culture, particularly when they do not share the beliefs and values of the mental health system we represent.

Josie Lomax

Josie Lomax lives alone in a private house. She retired from being a legal secretary several years ago. She had been working part time and had been feeling very tired at the time of her retirement, but now she misses the social aspects that work had for her, and is feeling that her life is lacking direction. This is exacerbating the low moods she has, and she is worried she is getting depressed again. She was diagnosed with clinical depression in her early 30s soon after she got divorced. Since that time, she has had a number of periods of depression, one of which required admission to hospital. Recently, she discussed with her GP that she no longer wanted to take the medication prescribed, as she had been on it so long that she did not know anymore what her 'normal' was, and she had struggled with side effects over the years. The GP has not been encouraging with this and has suggested that she try a new medication that may not have the same adverse effects for her.

On a one-to-one basis while discussing her mental health problems, how will you promote Mrs Lomax's mental health in relation to ensuring

- respect and dignity?
- her right to be treated in a humane way?

An initial reaction to this scenario may be to decide that what she needs is help to adapt to her retirement, and increase her social contacts that are available in her local community, an approach that would be supported by findings in the Age Concern and Mental Heath Foundation (2005) research. This may very well be part of a solution, but there are other issues to be considered. Josie has grown older with a diagnosis of clinical depression, and could be referred to as a 'graduate', a term that is sometimes used to refer to someone who has grown older with a mental illness. As someone who was diagnosed maybe 30+ years ago with a mood disorder, Josie falls into a group of people whose needs have not been investigated. Policies have excluded or overlooked people such as Josie, and medical research has tended to focus on the disabling effects of schizophrenia over a lifetime. However, the increase in recent years of discussions of the 'recovery' approach, especially as the voice of the service user begins to be heard, provides an approach that may be more helpful and meaningful to the service user. Service-user groups are fighting back against the disabling effects of labelling and stigma of psychiatric diagnosis that create barriers between the diagnosed and the rest of the world, and attempting to change the focus of how mental ill health is understood, with an emphasis on equality, citizenship and social inclusion as a solution to improving well-being. However, little discussion specifically considers this in relation to older adults. Is this indirect discrimination at work again? Jane has clearly contributed to society as a citizen and clearly has many strengths, including managing her own illness for more than 30 years and maintaining employment. Mental health assessments often fail to focus on strengths, and even when they attempt to include this consideration, identifying these is often secondary and incidental to collecting information about interpreting symptoms for a medical diagnosis and providing medication. This is particularly true for older adults, who are more likely to receive pharmacological interventions rather than psychological. Thinking within a recovery framework such as this could be the most helpful approach. This would include an acceptance that she can think through her own decision about medication, and you could provide the information and support she needs to think through her options.

The decision-making matrix shown in Table 5.4 may be a useful tool to assist Josie. It illustrates the findings of a European study that investigated inner conflict of taking medication of 164 people (average age 40) diagnosed with schizophrenia (Robson 2005), though the findings shown could easily depict what Josie might say. The philosophy behind this was that choosing to take and stop medication is normal and expected, and this acceptance led to a reported loss of uncertainty about taking medication. There is no reason why this approach cannot be used with people in older age groups and with any diagnosis (one might question why so many research studies of this nature exclude over-65s). It aims to explore value people place on each of the good things and not so good things about taking medication.

Essentially, any helpful approach to Josie requires that her strengths are identified and acknowledged, an approach often not considered for older adults, particularly those with mental health problems. As Perkins and Tice (1995) note, 'the labelling of problems distinguishes people with problems from those without …', and '… it is difficult to support the dignity and worth of people

Table 5.4 Decision-making matrix

Taking medication	Not so good	Good
List your thoughts	• Side effects; tired, slow, weight gain • Fear of damage/dependence • Discomfort from route of administration • Poor symptom control • Stigma	• Improve symptoms; sleep, memory, aggression, physical feelings • Calmer • Control • Quality of relationships improved • Get on with life • Get back to work
Stopping taking medication	**Good**	**Not so good**
List your thoughts	• Stop side effects • Increased autonomy • Nothing • Less stigmatising	• Symptoms return • Going back to hospital • Losing autonomy and positive things in life • Losing the calmness e.g. 'things in the kitchen get louder and more noticeable'

along with the belief in individual and collective strength, while in the process of assessing liabilities' (pp. 85–86).

Patrick O'Sullivan

Patrick lives alone in a semi-detached house in a quiet suburb in a town in Manchester. He is a very single-minded person and has always prided himself on being self-sufficient through his 85 years of life. He is good friends with his neighbour, who has been helping him out recently, as Patrick's behaviour has changed. He has stopped going out and sometimes complains that this is due to the 'sinister men who keep hanging around on his path'. He has called the police a few times, but they have been unable to find any evidence of this group of men intimidating people. In addition, Patrick has said that he has started to see his little sister in the house (she died in a drowning accident when Patrick was 10 years old; she was 6). He is glad to see her and thinks that the time may have come for them to be together again.

Write down your responses to the following questions:

• How do you understand what is happening to Patrick?
• How significant do you think his childhood experiences are in the present time?

It is not difficult to establish a link between what would be described as 'psychosis' and his experience of tragedy and grief. Indeed, some may prefer to understand this entirely as a bereavement issue or a 'maladaptive' bereavement reaction. The practicalities of such a scenario may in fact lead to utilising mental health act legislation. However, despite this, when considering what will help and support Patrick, he cannot be lost behind the system and the stigma that comes with any diagnosis and detention.

As Patrick has led a full and successful life, it is easy to dismiss his childhood experience as a long time in the past and irrelevant to his current situation. However, in order to help and support Patrick, it may be necessary to understand what happened at the time of the accident when he was 10. There is some evidence to suggest that it is much more likely that experiences from childhood are influential in developing mental ill health in later life, than recent experience. For example, Kraaij and DeWilde (2001) found a strong association between the number of negative events in childhood and depression in later life; similarly, Ong and Carter (2001) discuss a case study that illustrates this. This goes back to understanding people, rather than the reductionist approach that assessment tools can encourage. Talking about the circumstances and effects of this experience and discussing it (rather than a one-way asking and answering of questions characteristic in assessments) is arguably central to helping Patrick now.

Conclusion

This chapter has explored some issues around possible individual perspectives. It raises questions about how we can best help people, that sometimes may feel in conflict with the requirements and pressures to acquire certain kinds of information for the 'job' or system. These two do not necessarily have to be in conflict, as it is the *how* we do things that needs the most consideration. It may be possible to meet many requirements of the 'job' without helping people at all (even though we believe we are), as reflected in one of the carer's comments. We can choose to do this, or we can reconsider what we are actually achieving for the clients and reflect on the kind of mental health practitioner we actually want to be.

Acknowledgements

I thank the Central Manchester Alzheimer's Society carers' support group, Joe McShane, Hugh Rae, mental-health nursing students at Salford University, Celeste Foster and Juliet Monk

Resources

http://www.rcpsych.ac.uk/ Royal College of Psychiatrists. Mental health information.
http://www.alzheimers.org.uk Support for people with dementia their families and carers
www.mentalhealth.org.uk Mental Health foundation. Search 'later life' – choose 'adults in later life with mental health problems' – choose 'additional resources' – choose 'my story'.

http://www.npcuk.org/briefings/B21healthcare.doc National pensioners convention report
http://www.kingsfund.org.uk/resources/publications/age.html Kings Fund publication. 'Age discrimination in health and social care'
http://www.mhilli.org mental health in later life UK inquiry
http://www.dh.gov.uk/assetRoot/04/06/72/47/04067247.pdf Implementing medicines-related aspects of the national service framework for older people
http://www.sign.ac.uk/pdf/sign86.pdf Scottish intercollegiate guidelines network, management of patients with dementia
http://www.csip.org.uk case services improvment partnership
http://www.mind.org.uk Mind mental health charity – see 'Access all ages' campaign
http://www.equip.nhs.uk/langwmids.html A comprehensive collection of resources for different health and related issues including access for refugees and asylum seekers to health and social support information in other languages.
http://www.fordementia.org.uk/
http://www.guidance.nice.org.uk/cg42/niceguidance/pdf/english

References

Age Concern and Mental Health Foundation (2005) *Things to Do Places to Go Promoting Mental Health and Well Being in Later Life*. London, Age Concern and the Mental Health Foundation.

Alzheimer's Society Newsletter (2005) Issue Number 20, April, London, Alzheimer's Society, p. 2.

Beckman, N., Waern, M. and Skoog, I. (2005) Determinants of sexuality in 70 year olds. *International Psychogeriatrics* **17** (supplement 2), 140.

Coyne Plum, K. (1987) How patients view recovery, what helps what hinders. *Archives of Psychiatric Nursing* **1** (4), 285–293.

Department of Health (2003) *Confidentiality. NHS Code of Practice*. London, Department of Health. http://www.dh.gov.uk/assetRoot/04/06/92/54/04069254.pdf

Gilchrist, P. (1999) *Turning Your Back on Us Older People and the NHS*. London, Age Concern.

Kraaij, V. and DeWilde, E. J. (2001) Negative life events and depressive symptoms in the elderly; a life span perspective. *Aging and Mental Health* **5** (1), 84–91.

Macleod, M. (1994) It's the little things that count; the hidden complexity of everyday clinical nursing practice. *Journal of Clinical Nursing* **3** (6), 361–368.

Marwaha, S. and Livingstone, G. (2002) Stigma racism or choice. Why do depressed ethnic elders avoid psychiatrists. *Journal of Affective Disorders* **72** (3), 257–265.

Ong, Y. L. and Carter, P. (2001) Grand rounds; I'll knock elsewhere – the impact of past trauma in later life. *Psychiatric Bulletin* **25** (11), 435–426.

Perkins, K. and Tice, C. (1995) A strengths perspective in practice. Older people and mental health challenges. *Journal of Gerontological Social Work* **23** (3/4), 83–97.

Robson, D. (2005) Ambivalence to antipsychotics – coexisting positive and negative thoughts (inner conflict). Institute of psychiatry. Paper presented at the *11th International Network for Psychiatric Nursing Research Conference (RCN)*, Oxford, 2005.

Walker, G., Starren, E. and Warner, J. (2005) Sexual activity and experience of management of sexual difficulties in older people with mental illness. *International Psychogeriatrics* **17** (supplement 2), 140.

Chapter 6
Legal and Ethical Frameworks for Mental Health Nursing

Michael Tullett

Introduction

Older people with mental health needs are among the most marginalised section of the community and, for the last decade, have been within the focus to develop an effective ethical approach to care. This chapter will argue that ethics have been seen to be the domain of professional strata set above practice and, as such, have been approached in a political or macroscopic manner. Recent international studies have been focused more upon the details surrounding individual care in an effort to understand why circumstances are as they are. This fits with the nursing approach and may offer a more acceptable route to an ethical framework for the future. The chapter aims to offer guidance in developing a practical approach to ethical dilemmas and provoke new thinking in those who have recently joined the ranks of professional carers.

There may be two ways in which we can see our involvement in care. In the first, we may feel we need to meet the biological needs of our patients and that in doing so, we will achieve a positive state. We may look at the way a person copes with illness and the changes this illness has brought to their life. In achieving the most stable physiological state possible, we may expect that the person will respond in a positive manner. An example may be a person with an infection behaving in a confused and bewildered manner. Once the infection is cured, the person's behaviour returns to normal. This follows a philosophical approach where the idea is of human nature being the result of biophysical structures. In philosophical terms, this situation is termed Cartesian rationality. The argument seeks to explain what human nature is and whence it derives.

However, it may be that the person with an infection is behaving in an irrational manner that is not totally the result of infection but of any number of converging circumstances. There may be no acceptable explanation for their behaviour in biological terms. Why does one person respond to infection in an agitated and confused manner, while another becomes withdrawn? These questions need further study to bring about some understanding of the person. The way in which we undertake such an understanding is the basis of an alternative philosophical approach where the methods we use to understand behaviour are more important than our putting a label upon it. This is the approach of

Foucault (1926–1984), a philosopher who rejects the quest for identifying what human nature is and seeks to demonstrate ways in which human nature may be studied. These two aspects set up the discussion of whether we are the product of our environment (Cartesian rationality) or the architects of our environment (Foucault).

Taking the approach that we do have an influence on our environment, it is clear that this influence changes as we learn and experience certain events. In care terms, as patients learn more about their own illness, so they rely less upon health-care staff to support them and take more self-directed activity based upon their own experiences and desires. Foucault calls this maturity. Put simply, the view is that as we come to understand our environment, so we are increasingly released from the confines of authority (Rabinow, 1991) which, in care terms, results in more self-care. This line of thinking does require us to recognise the pitfalls in that if we make decisions that are beyond our understanding, the outcome may result in additional problems. If we are to follow our own lines of reason, we must recognise our limitations and recognise the freedom of others to follow their own line of action. To assist us in this, we develop some quite complex psychosocial concepts.

These concepts help us to catalogue aspects of our environment. They act as a short-hand that allows decision-making to be both timely and easy. These concepts include *homogeneity*, which gives reference to predictable responses within a defined cohort. For example, youngsters who wear hooded jackets are *homogenised* by society as hooligans. The concepts also include *systematicity*, which may be read as the manner in which we enquire, become involved and are influenced by events. Our *system* of arriving at an outcome contains set moves which in nursing may be identifying health needs through assessment, planning care, implementing this care and evaluating the results. Finally, we develop *generality*, which acts to make sense of events and influences in our lives. We *generalise* the health needs of older people, often leaning toward age being synonymous with frailty and ill health.

These concepts become the rule, allowing us to focus upon the further development of our own lines of action and demand no further exploration in most cases. They become the environment or context in which we act and expect others to interact.

Contexts and circumstances

This chapter is about identifying and upholding the moral entitlements of older people with mental health needs, and it is necessary to identify both the philosophical context and the care circumstances before seeking ethical processes and outcomes. Johnstone (1999) states that special attention is warranted in the area of mental health as it is seen to be an area neglected in mainstream bioethics discourse. People with mental health needs are the most stigmatised, discriminated against, marginalised, disadvantaged and hence vulnerable people in society, with societal attitudes of fear, ignorance and intolerance continuing to support the status. Current common law lacks consistency, and people's autonomy is not always respected. People can be written off as incapable because of a mental health diagnosis, and there is no clear legal authority for people who act on behalf of a person lacking mental capacity. There are limited options for people who want to plan ahead for loss of mental capacity and no right for relatives and carers to be consulted (Department of Constitutional Affairs, Department of Health, Public Guardianship Office, Welsh Assembly Government, 2005). Wider issues include restrictions on eligibility for insurance and superannuation schemes, employment and education and training (Johnstone, 1999).

Groups at risk – complexities

In relation to older people, there are two groups for whom challenges exist. In the first are those who have had enduring or severe mental health needs throughout adulthood, and in the second are those who develop 'age-associated' mental illness through the onset of frailty or dementia.

The World Psychiatric Association (1997) identified the complexity of disciplines working with these groups of older people; they note intricate problems not only to mental health and behaviour, but also to physical health and relational, environmental, spiritual and social matters. It is widely accepted that older people do experience increased incidences of physical illness, especially as they reach the eighth and ninth decades of life, and the current socio-medical focus demands that there be a holistic approach to care. The situation of care is closely linked to the family's customs and cultures, alongside the organisation of public health and social care demanding a blend of multiple services to meet the person's needs. Within our society today, unprecedented family change has taken place with four generation families becoming common, and increasing multi-cultural and ethnic diversity represented in the vast majority of local communities. The organisation of care needs to develop and maintain a focus on the patient and the family, and yet integrate into medical and social networks in such a way as to deliver specific and competent care. Competency has become the byword for services with the threat of culpability and legal liability as a constant reminder to maintain professionalism.

The need for an ethical framework

The Fifty-Fifth World Health Assembly of the World Health Organisation identified the need for guidance in developing comprehensive mental health care services in the prevention, early diagnosis and intervention in the management of mental health conditions for older people (World Health Organisation, 2002). In October 2002, the Royal College of Psychiatrists defined good practice in the management of people who enter old age and who suffer enduring mental health conditions. The major mental health conditions were seen to be chronic schizophrenia and relapsing mood disorders (Royal College of Psychiatrists, 2002). The Royal College of Psychiatrists has estimated that 11–60 per 100 000 of the national population are severely affected by chronic schizophrenia and/or relapsing mood disorders, many of whom exhibit florid symptoms (Royal College of Psychiatrists, 2002). Mental capacity issues potentially affect everyone, with over two million people in England and Wales lacking mental capacity to make some decisions for themselves (Department of Constitutional Affairs, Department of Health, Public Guardianship Office, Welsh Assembly Government, 2005). These include people with dementia, learning disabilities, mental health conditions, stroke and head injuries, with up to 6 million informal carers, social care and health-care professionals who may provide care or treatment for them (Department of Constitutional Affairs, Department of Health, Public Guardianship Office, Welsh Assembly Government, 2005). There is unlikely to be a family within the UK that has not been touched by mental illness in one form or another.

There have then been a number of triggers for review of the services provided to older people with mental health needs over the past decade, but Horsfall and Cleary (2002) note that projects to bring about such improvements lack a substantial ethical focus. They call for closer links between ethics and quality improvements through the provision of ethical guidelines.

Codes of conduct as ethical components

The scope of ethics relating to care and treatment is often based on professional codes of conduct, with the relationship between ethics and law being considered at a level set above practice, noticeably through the work of Ethics Committees. Topics considered by these committees are largely based upon the welfare of the public, the individual and organised professional activity. As such, there is less focus upon the individual than there would be where considerations were made at the practitioner level.

In terms of those with mental health conditions, legal pressure is applied to protect the public from violent assault. Where a person has a mental health condition and is potentially or actually a threat to others, the law overrules the principle of autonomy in the interests of the masses. The reasons are sound, but the outcome is dependent upon allegations made and the justification that results – the stronger the allegation, the louder the justification for overruling autonomy. Recent media reports strongly support the continual detention of people purely on the basis of being diagnosed with a major psychiatric condition.

In seeking to establish a pragmatic approach to decision-making in the provision of care for older people with mental health conditions, the client's interest is most often key. However, this is not always as clear as first thought. Codes of conduct do not always provide for the welfare of the patient, and the spectre of 'who pays' frequently drives the process. A tripartite occurs here – the professional is obliged to uphold their professional code of conduct, the purchaser is obliged to achieve best value and the patient may claim the moral right to their say and expect that to be upheld.

The politics of society vs. the individual

Edgley et al. (2006) note mental health practice has 'become the archetypal arena in which the political philosophical tensions between the rights of the individual and the rights of the community are played out'. The care vs. control argument continues in the mental health care arena fuelled by inquiry outcomes that mirror catalogues of failure and inadequate protection of the public. The Clunis inquiry (Court, 1994, p. 613) identified the demand to base future care management on past behaviours, '… patient's past behaviour should be used to predict likely future behaviour'. It is argued that generalisation has occurred with attitudes toward all mental illness coming to accept the loss of autonomy in people who face issues of decisional capacity as a result of mental health deficits in old age.

How do services enable clients?

There are distinctions made as to the welfare and interests of patients in terms of rights of access to an appropriate service. These distinctions will depend upon available resources across the public, voluntary and private sectors. Older people with mental health needs who find themselves institutionalised commonly experience care that is limited through a systematic approach that lacks resources (reflecting Foucault's *systematicity*). Resources in this case may include adequately trained and sufficient numbers of staff and well-defined care interventions. In the event of an individual being offered care where options are based upon limited resources, it may be difficult to support a claim that this is in their best interests. However, in circumstances where the person refuses care, the concept of best interest is frequently adopted to counter the refusal.

For example, an older gentleman who is confused and active may seek to leave the care area to attend his perceived workplace or some other activity associated with his past. The care service may be limited in the number of staff available and in the skills and knowledge those staff have to manage the situation. The solution or care intervention, may be to reduce his activity through chemical means. As a result of taking medication to reduce his wandering, the man develops a real risk of falling while mobilising. This risk is countered through the use of increased physical restraint. The gentleman becomes dissatisfied with the situation and finds, when he refuses medication or to sit where he is told, that he is confronted with the rationale that this is all in his best interest. It could be said the patient is condemned to accept what is offered rather than what is best practice. It could also be said that he has had his rights removed through a service that is failing to meet his needs. Conversely, it may also be considered whether or not it is reasonable to claim a right to something that does not exist, even if the reason is based in the financial and business priorities of the service provider. If the resources paid for do not enable the care team to offer a Gold-Standard service, it must be asked whether it is reasonable to expect such service. It may be of value to reflect upon the philosophical issues here. Are we, as nurses, the product of our environment and helpless in the face of organisational power, or are we the architects of the circumstances?

The argument of best interest

Where arguments of best interest occur, they are frequently accompanied by ensuring that ethical considerations are applied to avoid exposure to excessive or unnecessary risk. The identification of risk often acts as the basis upon which the relationships and communication processes develop between patients and professionals (British Medical Association, 2004). Professionals hold status that provides an advantage in decision-making within patient and professional interactions. The concept of 'Doctor knows best' remains a strong public perception. This concept in the establishment of 'best interest' is arrived at by analysing value-based judgements. This analysis is largely drawn from:

- making comparisons with other experiences;
- clarifying key concepts in the approach to care; and
- developing a logical line of action.

For example, the gentleman above who is active, is at risk of falling, and suffers cognitive impairment is a familiar situation to those working with people suffering dementia. There are plenty of past experiences with which to make comparisons. The key concepts may be seen as the likelihood of injury to the person and, it must be said, closely followed by the requirement for high levels of staff involvement in the event of him requiring post-injury care. The logical action may be to restrict the person's activity, thereby reducing the likelihood of further falls.

This is indisputable logic, but there are other factors to consider. The gentleman may be unable or unwilling to accept such restrictions, and there is no clear process to determine jointly agreed safe restrictions. In these circumstances, it is almost inevitable that the communication processes between professionals and the patient become confrontational, with poor consequences to the therapeutic relationship. In order to rectify this situation, it is important to return to the first premise: to what extent is the occurrence of falls with this individual really comparable with the falls experienced by others?

There are other factors to be investigated before committing to a superficial and what may be seen to be an organisationally convenient view. The use of hypnotic or sedative medications is overwhelmingly identified to be precursors to serial falls and must be considered in association with other acute or chronic central-nervous-system changes. We need to consider the potential presence of infections and the extent to which mobility deficits may be made more deficient through enforced reduced activity. Having made these considerations, are the key concepts valid in this case, or are they generalised concepts that act to support the manner in which the establishment operates? If it is considered that the organisation may only deal with this in its procedurally prescribed manner, the risk is that staff duty rotas will drive variable approaches. When sufficient staff are 'on duty', one approach may be used, but when less staff are available, another approach is required. The maintenance of the person's autonomy will be lost in the search for corporate safety.

Unless key concepts include the person at the centre, it is likely that activity will revolve around the routine and needs of the establishment. This is a whisker away from the removal of human rights and has been seen to result in people being physically and/or chemically restrained as a considered response to risk, and even as an argued ethical response to the situation. This does identify superficial ethical actions that are potentially harmful, a situation it would be reasonable to avoid.

At this point, it may be helpful to review some ethical principles and look at some of the ethical frameworks used in this area of care.

Current ethical frameworks

In order to make valued decisions relating to care, there needs to be an acceptable framework upon which decisions may be formulated and checked against. The most commonly used ethical model is that described by Beauchamp and Childress (2001) in which the principles of autonomy (respecting the decision-making capacities of the autonomous person, enabling individuals to make reasoned and informed choices), beneficence (the balance of the benefits against the risk and costs, the profession acts in such a way as to benefit the person), nonmaleficence (avoiding causing harm or ensuring the degree of harm caused by treatment is minimal and not disproportionate to the benefits of treatment) and justice (distributing benefits risks and costs fairly). The notion is the person in similar situations will be treated in a similar fashion. This model has close associations with both medical and legal aspects of care and acts to underpin central themes of Human Rights in promoting autonomy as the primary principle upon which actions are measured. Other principles may be overruled by the demand for autonomy, demonstrating the linear approach to the model. Based upon Hippocratic principles, this has become the bio-ethic model of choice, but there are questions raised as to its adequacy in nursing.

Different disciplines in health and social care may adopt different frameworks. Tschudin (2005) demonstrates this in describing the work of Gilligan whereby ethics need relativity to the work undertaken by a specific professional group. In nursing, the relationship between the nurse and the client centres upon emotions, affections and other significant relationships in the client's life, requiring specific attitudes and skill sets in decision-making. Such decisions require the needs of the person to be heard, and the response is often described as intuitive rather than pragmatic. Manning (1998) describes five elements for ethics in nursing: moral attention, sympathetic understanding, relationship awareness accommodation and response. Roach (1992) describes another framework she terms the 'Five C's', in which Compassion, Competence, Confidence, Conscience, and Commitment are the basis of developing ethical care. In these approaches, time is needed to take less of a linear view and more of a personal view that recognises the existence and the content of meaningful relationships in the person's life. The result of this perspective is the development of a logical response with steps that are drawn from the individual's account of illness and loss of well-being.

It is reasonable to suggest that the nursing ethics are not as powerful in society as the biomedical approach. International efforts are being undertaken to establish a framework for ensuring the protection of the moral entitlements of people with mental health conditions. In Australia, efforts to develop such a framework focus upon the education of the public, on identifying mental-health promotion strategies and upon developing preventative mental health programmes that clarify risk-management strategies and are based in research activity. It is their intention to develop a substantive mental health-care ethical framework based upon human rights. This work follows on from the recognition of the need for protection against abuse and neglect, and the United Nations General Assembly (1991) adopted Principles for 'The protection of person's with Mental Illness and for the Improvement of Mental Health Care'. The Australian model of mental health care ethics proposes that all people should expect and be provided with:

- adequate access to high-quality and culturally appropriate mental health-care services;
- circumstances to make informed choices about care and treatment;
- privacy, dignity and respect;
- being treated fairly;
- mechanism of complaint and redress;
- advocacy;
- legislation that affirms their fundamental rights;
- review of mental health legislation, updated as necessary;
- access to relatives and friends;
- rehabilitation;
- the right equal to other citizens to health care, income maintenance, education, employment, housing, transport, legal services, equitable health and other insurance and leisure appropriate to one's age.

The model continues further to note: 'The diagnosis of mental health problems or mental disorder is not an excuse for inappropriately limiting their rights' (Mental Health Consumer Outcomes Task Force, Australia, 1995).

Nursing is a profoundly moral activity based upon the development of relationships and processes of therapeutic intervention. Under this model, the relationships involved must be looked at in detail. Responsibilities for people who have mental health needs include to 'respect the human worth and dignity of other people; and to participate as far as possible in reasonable treatment and rehabilitation processes' (Mental Health Consumer Outcomes Task Force, 1995).

Whose right and whose duty?

The dilemma arising from this is based upon the need to accept moral rights in doing one's duty. In relation to the gentleman considered earlier who is falling, it may be argued that he has a personal, moral duty to maintain his own safety. If he refuses treatment, he may claim the moral right and expect that right to be upheld now consider to what extent he is carrying out his own personal duty when making such a refusal.

The practitioner is ultimately bound to accept the patient's right of refusal, even though, from the practitioner's perspective, the outcome may not be in the patient's best interest. The responsibility of the practitioner is to ensure that such a decision is made with adequate and appropriate information. Serious questions may arise where there is a perception that through refusing treatment, the patient will increase their suffering and act with increased risk to others. Even more questions are raised where risks are identified by professionals but not even recognised by the person they look after.

To give an example, we may return to our gentleman who is active and confused. The identification of risk is a professional outcome, based upon the experience of caring for others. The man himself has no concept of this risk and subsequently fails to share the recognition that any change in behaviour is required. The role for professionals in this case is to establish a method of communication that facilitates the recognition of the likelihood of his falling. Manning's (1998) elements of ethical care may be a useful framework to use in this case.

According to Manning, it is important to seek the details of need. This man has a point he wishes to make, and it is our ethical duty to seek clarity and develop an understanding of this point. He believes he has obligations to meet elsewhere, and it is our role to identify these obligations and offer a safe passage to his achieving the demands he sees are upon him. This does not mean we are colluding with some delusional state but that we recognise the importance of his behaviour to him and spend time exploring them. We approach this in such a way as to identify with him. We need to find what demands he feels are made upon him and what priorities may be established that are acceptable to him. Initially, there is a bond between 'fellow creatures' that enables us to develop awareness of other needs (in this case, the need to meet obligations and maintain safety in mobilising). In working in a collaborative way, we enable the man to explore his sense of self and to recognise other priorities, which may include his duty of care to himself. This meets with Manning's relationship awareness. Finally, the manner in which this communication takes place is between the client and the professional, a relationship that needs to take account of power ratios.

Who has the ultimate answers, and who will make the final decision? This takes us back to the Foucault principles at the beginning of the chapter: are we enabling maturity or are we supporting a paternalistic state? Time is required to ensure that the power is with the client and that decisions are agreed. This process will offer accommodation of the client's needs and act to sustain care in the future. Successful negotiations may be reused in full or in part to support future areas of difficulty. The incident then becomes a part of the dynamic relationship that acts to identify the client and the professional as partners.

The use of advocacy

A common adjunct in the situation above is the use of an advocate. This may be seen to be an advantage where a relative or significant other person in the patient's life is co-opted to establish concordance with a risk strategy. However, this does carry risks of its own. Although perhaps attractive in a practical sense there are two aspects to consider. What real authority does another person have to demand concordance to care and what will be the impact of using such authority upon the individual and his well-being? If the individuals feel their autonomy has been taken by another, the consequences will be that the individual loses self-image and self-esteem. Outside the individual, it must also be considered whether another person has the right to take on such a role where individual rights may be abdicated and passed to another. The role of advocacy does require context to ensure that the rights of one group (society and the professional 'duty of care') are not in conflict or competition with the rights of the individual. Advocacy needs to focus upon assisting the patient to recognise the risk and not upon changing behaviour through developing and applying emotionally charged sanctions.

Moral or civil rights?

One major consideration of care provision is how activity is meeting legislation. Legal cases, based upon civil liberties, make decisions where institutional care is provided against the person's will. Most often, this arises where there is perceived risk posed by and/or to the individual. The balance in assessing whether or not the actions of the individual are seen to be a substantial risk is influenced by the requirement to support the individual's civil liberty. Unless there is clear cause for removing the person's liberty, the risks posed will not influence the decision. An example of this may be seen where a patient lacks the capacity to make decisions as a result of cognitive loss. Our older gentleman who is at risk of falling may refuse assistance to wash and dress or, in a domiciliary setting, refuse carer's access to his home. There is no shared contact upon which to develop Manning's care elements, and the service is left powerless to intervene without access to a court order. The legal demand is for proof that he is at risk. There are inherent difficulties here, and until the man has suffered as a result of falling or self-neglect to a degree that identifies this as 'previous behaviour', the degree of proof is unlikely to sway a decision for formal admission under the Mental Health Act 1983. The Human Rights approach to ethics in mental health care is then quite problematic. Not only do the rights of different people conflict, but when applied to the scope of available care and to the legal system, there is concern over what is a moral right and what a civil right is.

The area of practical ethics in mental health care must encompass the broad moral issues. Quite apart from the politically adopted issues of competency, privacy and consent, practice ethics must focus upon the mutuality, the therapeutic alliance, safety, security, trust, compassion and empathy, which are imperatives of the professional–client relationship (Johnstone, 1999). There must be a focus upon the consequences of stigma and discrimination and the transcultural nature of mental health care.

Johnstone (1999) offered such a focus in describing key issues identified by people with mental health conditions as:

- the desperate need for understanding;
- the need to speak openly and be heard;
- the longing for acceptance by others of the mystery and the unpredictability of their illness;
- the desire to be equal with others.

There are difficulties in an acute psychiatric setting where timeliness of treatment may be critical. There is a likelihood of these issues becoming swamped by the urgency of the situation. In this case, there needs to be some planning.

Advanced directives

One approach in supporting an effective ethical approach is the Advanced Directive or Advanced Statement. The occurrence of serious mental illness may be accompanied by a lack of concordance with effective treatment approaches. At a time of serious illness, with accompanying risks of self-harm or harm to others, it is medically imperative that treatment be provided speedily and effectively. This brings the risk of these people having medical treatments imposed upon them, against their will. It is argued that such imposition may compound feelings of distress and produce feelings of violation in the sufferer, close companions and even witnesses.

The application of an advanced directive would allow the individual to state what approaches are best suited to their moral interests, welfare and well-being, in the event of them requiring acute psychiatric intervention at a time in the future. In the event of such a directive being invoked, the post-acute phase of illness should be a time to review the directive and update or confirm acceptable treatment options in the event of a further episode of illness. This is formalised in the Mental Capacity Act 2005.

The Mental Capacity Act, 2005

The application of an Advanced Directive would start the process by offering a valid history from which to begin negotiations. The principles of such a contract are provided by the Department of Health (2005) and consist of allowing an individual to refuse specified medical treatment in advance. They are legally binding now, but the Act gives greater safeguards requiring that they must be made when the person has capacity, and comes into effect if they subsequently lack capacity. The Act is very precise and requires clarity about which treatment it applies to and when. It must be in writing and witnessed if it applies to life-sustaining treatment. Even so, doctors can provide treatment if they have any doubt that the advance decision is valid and applicable.

The principles of the Mental Capacity Act 2005 assume that a person has capacity unless proved otherwise. It requires that services do not treat people as incapable of making a decision unless all practicable steps to help them have been tried, and it does not allow treatment to be enforced solely because their decision appears unwise. The principles do rely upon the aspect of best interest but also require consideration of whether the outcome may be achieved in a less restrictive way, before doing something to someone or making a decision on their behalf.

In assessing capacity, the Act sets out the best practice approach to determining capacity, based upon whether an individual is able, at a particular time of making a particular decision. It is decision-specific, so the decision that a person lacks capacity to determine their place of abode does not automatically mean that they lack capacity to choose the food they eat, the clothes they wear or the activities they engage in throughout the day. Each of these elements would require a separate decision-making process, and the process is susceptible to scrutiny from the newly formed Public Guardianship Office. This area is closely linked to the issue of consent.

Consent

If a person is seen to lack capacity, no other person may provide consent for treatment relating to their needs. Again, the 'best interest' aspect is used in law, but these must include the previous wishes and beliefs of the individual, before they lost capacity, their current beliefs and wishes, their general well-being and their spiritual and religious welfare. This information is most often only available where a relative or significant person in their life is available to relay it, although in some cases, previous hospital admissions may contain relevant notes. Consent previously given may be withdrawn at any time, resulting in the need to consider very carefully what the consequences of refusal to consent may be and what the consequences of overriding the individual's autonomy would be in the event of adopting a 'best interest' approach.

Conclusion

To summarise, many of the issues explored are seen to derive from taking either the Cartesian rationality approach of Chomsky or the Foucaultian approach to the study of ethics. The biomedical ethics of Beauchamp and Childress (2001) are strong in distinguishing ethical processes but do not identify the elements of nursing, which demand a greater focus upon the relationship between professionals and users. However, since the early 1990s, international efforts have been ongoing to identify an ethical framework that will support people with mental health needs. It may be argued that the focus has been upon seeking to understand what elements of human nature need support and what elements should be restricted, which may be seen to be reflected in the demand to predict and manage areas of risk for the benefit of the public.

The emerging themes take a different perspective and, rather than seeking to identify elements of human nature, are more inclined to describing circumstances in which human nature may be either supported or threatened. In this way, the perception of best interest is based not only on risk but on the ability of the service to meet needs. It becomes clear that services are not omnipotent and frequently act in a self-supportive manner rather than an advocative manner. Service design is therefore paramount in achieving an ethical position in care provision.

There has been a great deal of emphasis upon regulation of care services with an expectation that such regulation will result in service improvement. The work in Australia is an example of this but the basis of this work is more set in the Foucault tradition than is seen in equitable work undertaken in Europe and the USA. The importance is in the detail, and the ethical process needs to be set at the practitioner level. We do face increasing legal pressure in our professional lives, and there is a requirement to manage the interface between care and the courts. The role of the Ethics Committee should be to make the distinction between moral and civil rights, but that should not detract from practitioners working to establish a client–professional relationship that is based upon sound ethical principles. Finally, the areas of capacity and consent need to be seriously considered on a case-by-case basis. There is no definitive ruling, and any legal proceedings will certainly seek the process used in arriving at individual decisions. A well-developed ethical approach that uses a recognised framework will assist the practitioner in developing a robust approach.

References

Beauchamp, T. and Childress, J. (2001) *Principles of Bio-Medical Ethics*, 5th edn. Oxford, Oxford University Press.

British Medical Association (2004) *Interface between the NHS and Private Treatment*. London, British Medical Association.

Court, C. (1994) Clunis inquiry cites 'catalogue of failures'. *British Medical Journal* **308**, 613.

Department of Constitutional Affairs, Department of Health, Public Guardianship Office, Welsh Assembly Government (2005) *Mental Capacity Act Summary* 2005. www.dca.gov.uk/legal-policy/mental-capacity/mca-summarypdf

Department of Health (2005) *Mental Capacity Act 2005.* www.dh.gov.uk/publications

Edgley, A., Stickley, T. and Masterson, S. (2006) Whose right? *Journal of Mental Health* **15** (1), 35–42.

Horsfall, J. and Cleary, M. (2002) Mental health quality improvement: What about ethics? *International Journal of Mental Health Nursing* **11** (1), 40–46.

Johnstone, M. (1999) *Bioethics: A Nursing Perspective*, 4th edn. Edinburgh, Churchill Livingstone.

Manning, R.C. (1998) A care approach. In: *A Companion to Bioethics* (H. Kuhse and P. Singer, eds). Oxford, Blackwell, pp. 98–105.

Mental Health Consumer Outcomes Task Force, Australia (1995) www.achs.au

Rabinow, P. (1991) *The Foucault Reader: An Introduction to Foucault's Thoughts.* Harmondsworth, UK, Penguin.

Roach, S. (1992) The aim of philosophical inquiry in nursing. Unity or diversity of thought. In: *Philosophic Inquiry in Nursing* (J. Kikuchi and H. Simmons, eds), pp. 38–44. Newbury Park, Sage.

Royal College of Psychiatrists (2002) Council Report: *Caring for People who Enter Old Age with Enduring or Relapsing Mental Illness ('Graduates')*. London, Royal College of Psychiatrists.

Tschudin, V. (2005) *Ethics in Nursing, The Caring Relationship*. London, Butterworth-Heinmann.

United Nations General Assembly (1991) The protection of person's with mental illness and for the improvement of mental health care. http://www.ohchr.org/english/law/olderpersons.htm

World Health Organisation (2002) *Regional Strategy for Mental Health; 52nd Session*, Brunie Darrussalem, 10–14 September 2001. Geneva, World Health Organisation.

World Psychiatric Association (1997) www.wpanet.org/home.html

Chapter 7
Dilemmas in Mental Health Nursing

Tina Naldrett

Introduction

Caring for older people with mental health needs can be a challenge. Sometimes they find themselves in places or with teams that do not traditionally have a background in caring for them. This chapter starts from the premise that we might all be challenged by the dilemmas of balancing older people's rights with management of risk, and it attempts to explore practical solutions.

One current dilemma concerns who is best to provide the care and support of older people at this time of need, identified by the *Living Well In Later Life* report (Commission for Healthcare Audit and Inspection, 2006). This criticises the way in which current NHS hospitals and care systems continue to fail older people by not ensuring they are in the right place, for the right care and treatment, at the right time.

The report states that 'some older people experience poor standards of care on hospital wards, including . . . being repeatedly moved from one ward to another for non-clinical reasons' and that ' the division between mental health services and older people has resulted in the development of an unfair system'. Many nurses working within that system want to offer the best possible evidence-based care and support. This can only aid older persons in their need for respect and a dignified therapeutic alliance with the people in whose care they find themselves (McCormack, 2005).

To begin, we will look at rights, risks and responsibilities, and how the care and support we give can sit within this framework to offer a balance between independence and safety. Some of the dilemmas in caring for and supporting older people with mental health needs will be identified and therapeutic approaches detailed. The abuse of older people will also be defined and the role of the nurse and the required actions discussed. Ethical frameworks have been discussed in Chapter 6. This chapter will explore further how person-centred ethical frameworks can assist in practice and will describe some practical measures for supporting older people.

Rights, risks and responsibilities related to restraint

Guidance from the Royal College of Nursing (2004) gives us the opportunity to open up some discussions about the use of restraint. Issues arise when we try to keep people safe while retaining their independence and maintaining a therapeutic alliance with them. Restraint is an emotive issue for all, and those working with older people need practical solutions, which respond to older people's complexity. The premise behind using any form of restraint is that it is a last option when all other therapeutic ways forward have been tried and have failed.

Restraint is described as an intervention which prevents a person from behaving in 'ways that threaten or cause harm, to themselves, others or to property' (Duff et al., 1996). Methods of restraint include:

- holding back;
- confinement to a chair, using a beanbag as a chair;
- keeping in bed with bed rails or using a mattress on the floor;
- keeping in a limited environment, e.g. a ward or room;
- withdrawal of sensory aids such as glasses;
- controlling language, non-verbal communication and body language;
- medication.

Care must be taken when using restraint. As highlighted by Watson (2005), even in situations where they feel that restraint is justified, staff may actually be abusing the person whether or not they are solving the problem. Restraint can be a symptom of busyness, of inadequate staffing or of the person being in the wrong environment. So, assessment is key in identifying the underlying cause and need for restraint.

Avoiding the use of restraint, assessing the risks

The assessment of risk is twofold:

- On one hand, the professionals and other significant people in the older person's life have to be prepared to take some risks to preserve their dignity and freedom. Carers can be quick to reduce people's choices and movements because they fear the outcome if they do not.
- On the other hand, we can avoid some use of restraint by assessing risks and planning their avoidance or management. For example, if Robert, an accountant and lifelong bachelor experiencing dementia, who has never liked baths or showers and has only ever stripped to wash, has been hitting out at care staff in the bathroom, it would be sensible to approach his hygiene needs with this in mind. Staff could offer a bowl for a wash or private time in the bathroom with a sink. Perhaps he would prefer a male carer, if possible? And will it make a great deal of difference if, on one difficult day, he does not

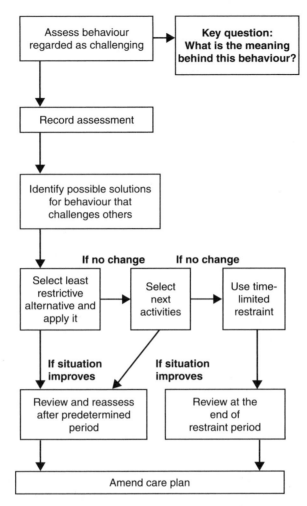

Fig. 7.1 Steps for approaching the risk of restraint. Reproduced with kind permission from the Royal College of Nursing (2004), *Restraint revisited – rights, risks and responsibility: Guidance for nursing staff.* London, RCN.

wash at all or until later when he is calmer? Sometimes it is the pressure of the hospital routine or other people's agendas that take control from older people.

The scheme for the implementation of restraint shown in Figure 7.1 shows the steps for approaching that risk assessment.

Our responsibility in relation to restraint

The nurse has a duty of care to the older person, The Nursing and Midwifery Councils Code of Professional Conduct (Nursing and Midwifery Council, 2004) states that in the care of a professional nurse, 'clients should be safe and respected as individuals whose interest and dignity are respected'. The use of restraint should be used within this duty of care. It should be planned, and any restraint used should be recorded, monitored and reviewed regularly, and so only used for the minimum of time needed.

If nurses are confronted with the dilemma of using restraint, they will need to decide how to act, using their professional knowledge and expertise to problem-solve ways forward. This offers an opportunity for us to work more closely with older persons and those significant in their life, along with the multi-disciplinary team and colleagues in mental health and social care to share perspectives that create a supportive plan of care (McCormack, 2005).

This calls for the nurse to make decisions and judgements as part of the assessment process (Taylor, 2005) using both rational thinking and their intuition, a useful skill when working with older people experiencing mental health problems who may try to communicate with us on many levels, and who will continue to want information and advocacy which keeps their sense of independence throughout any difficult times (Denning, 2005).

While outlining plans, the nurse should be aware that the employer as well as our professional body governs the decisions made. This means we have to be aware of, and act in line with, local policies and procedures that relate to restraint. Do you know what these are? It is worth checking good practice and policies where you work. To continue improving our practice, we can review care, reflect, carry out audits that compare our practice to others and keep ourselves in touch with the evidence base to make sure we respond in the best way we can for older people.

Older people's rights

When we set out to protect older people at all costs, we can compromise their rights. Consent is a basic right that belongs to the older person, and they can decide if they wish to walk around or to have a wash or not. Sometimes their decisions are not in line with what others want them to do, but they still have the right to make them. It is best practice to check out consent each time, just in case the person has changed their mind since you last cared for them (Department of Health, 2001). When adults give legal consent, they are described as competent and they may sign something, but if the consent was obtained in a way that they did not fully understand, it will not be valid.

Dilemmas in caring for and supporting older people with mental needs

- Ensuring that the older person continues to be seen as an individual when their behaviour is challenging or difficult to understand.
- Ensuring that the older person's mental health needs are assessed and identified correctly, even in settings where staff are not expert at this, so they receive the care, support and treatment they need.

- Keeping the older person themselves safe, while retaining their independence and ensuring they receive physical care, which will reduce any harm to their general well-being.
- Keeping others in the shared environment safe and respect everyone's rights.
- Identifying any abuse of the older person and ensuring that this is dealt with appropriately.
- Ensuring that the person's life history and a biographical approach is used when the older individual themself may not be able to reliably inform this.
- Working with older people with mental health needs in environments that are not designed to make that easy.
- Building a toolbox of skills and knowledge, which is current and can be utilised as the need arises when this is not part of a team's core knowledge or speciality.

When faced with decision-making in relation to these dilemmas, in order to protect the older person's best interests and maximise their potential for well-being, there will always be an ethical dimension. Every decision a nurse makes about an older person will need to consider their thoughts, wishes and desires (Melia, 2004; Nursing and Midwifery Council, 2004). In order to achieve this, nurses needs to remain objective and aware of their own feelings and assumptions in relation to the presenting situation. Sometimes it is helpful to undertake a check on our assumptions using the checklist in Table 7.1.

Having reviewed their assumptions, nurses will need to identify the issues relating to the decision or dilemma through a series of key questions which all relate to ethical decision-making:

- What is causing concern and to whom?
- What are the desired and realistic outcomes?
- What are the alternatives?
- Who feels obligations, and what are they?
- What beliefs and principles underpin what the older person thinks and what others think and believe about the situation.
- Who can and needs to make decisions?
- What has worked before?
- What has not worked before?
  Once we have worked through some of the key questions, we can look to the therapeutic approaches to see what might be helpful.

Some therapeutic approaches

Restraint is most commonly used to manage restless or agitated behaviour which, if left unchecked, could be dangerous to the person or others (Royal College of Nursing, 2004). By understanding and tackling the underlying cause, it might be possible to avoid using restraint. Offered here are some approaches that might help.

Table 7.1   Checklist of assumptions and helpful actions

Assumption checklist	Helpful actions
Am I anxious as a practitioner about my lack of required knowledge, and might it lead me to make a decision which could be better informed?	Recognise that this is OK. we all need to learn new things sometimes, seek help by talking to a mental health practitioner or someone with the knowledge you need, even if it means calling a neighbouring unit, another ward, or another home.
Do I fear the unknown, and what will happen?	The older person will be fearful of the unknown, too. Stay focused on clear assessment based on facts and what you observe. Begin to use essential communication skills to build a relationship which will help you both with a therapeutic connection (discussed further in Chapter 8).
Has the older person been labelled, and do they come to our service or my shift with a 'Bad Press'?	Look to the here and now: how does the older person appear to you at this moment? Sometimes, behaviour may have been erratic some time ago and has calmed now or may have been exaggerated by colleagues who need to build their own understanding of the older person with mental health needs.
Am I measuring this situation using past experience that did not go well?	If a past experience has left us feeling anxious about dealing with unusual behaviour, this may require some additional reflection to learn what we can do differently. Remembering that all experiences have their worth, use the past to inform this occasion with an open mind: this is a different person and circumstances, and the outcome will be different.

Checking the physical elements, a well-rounded approach

A physiological cause could be the reason behind a change in behaviour, and it is always worth checking through a list of possibilities. (Further discussion is offered in Chapter 14.)

Is the person experiencing:

- an adverse drug reaction?
- an infection, e.g. a urinary-tract infection or chest infection?
- dehydration?
- pain?
- restless legs from sitting a long time?
- constipation?
- malnutrition?
- poor sensory connection to the world due to lack of glasses or hearing aid?

They may be wandering because they are looking for their hearing aid, a drink, some exercise or the toilet. The drugs being used may need review for their side-effects or action on the older person, as often a smaller dose may be required, or multiple medicines may be interacting with one another (Levenson, 1998).

Using a biographical approach

Understanding the possible mindset of the older person with mental health needs can help nurses to relate to some of their behaviour, which in turn can help us to see why they might behave in certain ways and how we might help them if this leads to distress or a more general disruption in the care setting for themselves or others (Crump, 1998).

To help with this, I would like to introduce Glynis, who came to hospital in 2006. Here is a potted biography gained from conversations, her notes and a friend Mabel, who visits her at home three times a week. Understanding this approach and something of the person can enhance how nurses support them in an individualised way.

- 2006: Glynis came into hospital confused and disorientated; following a fall in the garden, she was there all day.
- 2002: Husband Ewan dies.
- 1992: Husband retires, and he and Glynis move to a seaside town.
- 1986: Son, aged 32 years, dies in a car accident.
- 1972: Daughter marries and has twins in the same year.
- 1956: Son, Bryn, is born.
- 1948: Daughter, Mary, is born.
- 1947: Glynis marries Ewan, a miner.
- 1927: Glynis is born, one of twins; twin dies.

Glynis may identify with the present or the past. If she has difficulty with her memory, which involves both the storage and retrieval of information, this may show in how she behaves. As memories often have feelings attached to them, she may seem irrational to others when, to herself, everything makes perfect sense for the time in which she currently sees herself. Looking at her history again, let us see how it could be from her point of view.

2006: Glynis came into hospital confused and disorientated

Glynis came into hospital confused and disorientated, following a fall in the garden, she was there all day. Glynis does not understand where she is, it hurts to urinate, her hip hurts, everyone is strange and it is very white and noisy. She thinks they have taken her purse and clothes away; where is Mabel? She feels abandoned and afraid, and will not let anyone take anything else away.

You can see how Glynis may not let others undress her, feels disempowered by the environment and the removal of her possessions for safe keeping and may not be clear in her communication about where she feels pain, so her hip problem and urinary-tract infection may go unnoticed.

2002: Husband Ewan dies

Glynis expected Ewan to die after his long illness, but she still feels the distress. She wants to cry in private. She wants to make sure he has a good send off.

He wanted to be buried, so there is a lot to do, and she will not leave it to others, so she cannot hang about here. It is making her so angry that she will get out and, if she has to, will sneak out.

If Glynis has taken herself back to this time, she may appear to be behaving irrationally, seeming to have a lot to organise. She is restless, not understanding where she is or the present time and is becoming upset and asking for family – perhaps Ewan, her husband (who you know to be dead) or her daughter, Mary?

1992: Ewan retires, and they move to seaside town

There is a lot to do with a new house to sort out. Glynis is well and busy looking forward to a new life by the sea. In her mind, Glynis may be in a place where she feels active and curious. Her behaviour might show the same thing; until she moves, she might forget she has hurt her hip, or has a urinary-tract infection or the limits of being in a hospital. She could think the hospital is a hotel where she is staying with Ewan until they move to the new house. Glynis may ask for him or speak of him as if he were around.

1986: Son dies in a car accident aged 32 years

Glynis still cannot believe Bryn has died. She cannot stop crying. She wants to visit the grave again, but when she left this place the other day, she did not even recognise the high street. What is wrong with everything, and why is she alone in this place? She is very afraid. She does not recognise anyone.

This may have been a very distressing time for Glynis. She may be tearful or asking for family. She may blame people, want to leave, and seem inconsolable, out of keeping with what is happening now. She may be in her memories when she did not live in the seaside town and may not recognise it as her home now.

1972: Daughter marries and has twins in the same year

Glynis feels so happy to have a wedding to organise and babies to look after. This is a lovely time, and she is knitting and making the cake, so there is a lot to do. She needs to see Mary again and sort out a few more bits. Where is Mary, and what is this place? When she asks you, she cannot get a straight answer.

This may be a busy, productive and happy time for Glynis; she may exhibit restlessness with lots on her mind. She may ask where the babies are and for Mary and the rest of her family. She may find reminders of the here and now annoying if she is fixed in 1972. In her mind, she is in her forties and could feel able and she may wonder why she is not as physically adept as she thinks she should be.

1956: has a son, Bryn

Having a baby is harder than people let on with an 8-year-old to look after as well. Glynis feels exhausted. Was that the baby crying again? She must go and see to it. Hopefully soon the blues will go, and she will feel a lot better.

Glynis may feel like a young woman who has small children. She may have suffered postnatal depression or struggled with the physical aspects of childrearing and housework in the 1950s. Her behaviour may mirror this tiredness. She could think she hears the baby and feel the urgency of having to attend to him.

1948: has a daughter, Mary

Glynis is enjoying the experience of being a first time Mum and has her own Ma around to help look after her daughter. She is 21 years of age and feels lucky to have her own place, a Miner's cottage and a husband who works hard for his family.

Glynis may see herself as a young woman with a busy life and responsibilities that she sees as important. She had her Ma helping her to raise her first child and may ask for her. This could make no sense to care staff if they are not aware that her memories may have taken her to this place.

1947: marries Ewan, a miner

Delighted to be marrying her childhood sweetheart who is a little older than her, Glynis thanks the Lord they survived the Second World War. New beginnings mean life is happy and hopeful. The wedding is on a shoestring, and she is helping Ma to make the dress and the cake.

A busy and hopeful time, with thrift in the post-war years, if her memory takes her to this time and place Glynis may present as distracted by her wedding plans and busyness.

Knowing a little of someone's biography cannot put us in their shoes. It can give us some insight into their behaviour and memories, allowing us to validate those feelings and need for activity. This allows the carer to acknowledge the feelings and emotions being experienced by the individual and accepts them without judgment (Feil 2002).

Using reality orientation

Helping someone to relate to the current reality can be helpful and is called orientation. However, when someone is confused, it can be very challenging to have someone constantly pointing out that you have a wrong idea of the time, the place you are in or who you are. Therefore, considerable skill is needed to communicate well using reality orientation. Twenty-four-hour reality orientation is good practice where the staff constantly remind people in natural conversation of the time, place and person

For example:

Nurse: 'Good morning. It's me, Nurse Clare. Is that the time, Edith, 10am? I don't know where the morning's gone. Would you like a mid-morning cup of tea or coffee?'
Edith: 'Yes, they say I have to drink. I'll have tea . . . have you seen my dad?'

Nurse: (knowing Edith's father to be dead) 'You must be thinking of your dad. Do you miss him? What was he like?'

Other therapies

Communication with older people is complex, especially as their mental health needs can lead them to be labelled and stigmatised as problem people (Crump, 1998). Therefore, any methods which connect with the inner person may be helpful. Advantages have been reported with the following dependent upon the individual need of the older person: music therapy, pet therapy, massage, aromatherapy, exercise and awareness of the environment (Phair, 1999).

Safeguarding adults

As discussed earlier, there is an inherent danger of blurring older people's restraint with 'elder abuse'. To prevent this from happening, it helps us to know about elder abuse. 'Safeguarding Adults' is a national framework outlining standards for good practice and outcomes in adult protection work (Association of Directors of Social Services, 2005). The definition of a vulnerable adult is a person aged 18 years or over: 'Who is or may be in need of community care services by reason of mental or other disability, age or illness; and who is or may be unable to protect him or herself against significant harm or exploitation' (Department of Health, 2000).

This definition starts to look at vulnerability, and what often makes older people vulnerable is abuse. This is an issue which can be fraught with conflict and awkwardness (Action on Elder Abuse, 2004; Manthorpe, 2005). However, as registered practitioners, we have a professional obligation to protect older people and to explore this area if abuse is suspected or stated (Nursing and Midwifery Council, 2004). Indeed, nurses are frequent referrers of incidents of abuse, as illustrated in a recent Department of Health audit (Department of Health, 2006).

What is abuse?

Abuse is defined by a user group as 'A single or repeated act or lack of appropriate action, occurring within any relationship where there is an expectation of trust, which causes harm or distress to an older person' (Action on Elder Abuse, 2006).

Abuse can be categorised into seven main categories:

- physical;
- sexual;
- psychological (including emotional abuse);
- financial;

- neglect/negligence;
- discriminatory;
- institutional.

A vulnerable adult can be (Department of Health, 2006):

- an adult to whom accommodation and nursing or personal care are provided in a care home;
- an adult to whom personal care is provided in their own home under arrangements made by a domiciliary care agency; or
- an adult to whom prescribed services are provided by an independent hospital, independent clinic, independent medical agency or National Health Service body.

Who are the abusers? Vulnerable adults may suffer abuse from a wide range of people. These can include relatives and family members, professional staff, carers, volunteers, neighbours, friends and other service users. Other abusers may be strangers or a person who deliberately targets a vulnerable person in order to exploit them. Consider the following situation, and how what you have read here about abuse may impact upon it.

Exploring a potential dilemma

Mr Evans has been caring for his wife, Pauline, with dementia for many years. Pauline has needed admission to her local care home for some time, as her management changes periodically, and Mr Evans needs time to plan and recoup his energies. This means that the team have known Pauline for 8 years or so now.

At the moment, Pauline does not speak and needs all physical care, which includes the monitoring and treatment of frequent urinary tract infections. The team feel, however, that they know her well enough to tell when she is happy or unhappy.

On this most recent admission, Mr Evans has decided that he can no longer care for her at home and is looking for a permanent place in a nursing home for her. However, he still comes to visit several times a week and on Sundays takes her home for lunch for a few hours.

When she returns, the staff say she is very agitated; she rocks in her chair, grinds her teeth and will not let the staff touch her to take off her cardigan. She settles within a few hours, but the staff are concerned and want to try and reduce her distress.

When discussing the way forward in a handover, several of the team members share that, when they take her to the toilet after she returns from the Sunday visits, they find her sticky with some sort of vaginal lubrication or secretion.

What might be the issues here? When looking at the situation, a team must be careful to explore all possibilities and steer clear of making assumptions. One would have to consider the possible reasons for Pauline's agitation. Could it be that she does not understand why she has to return to hospital following her visits home? Could it be that something uncomfortable or undesirable is happening to her on the visits home? Is there a way of gauging Pauline's ability to consent and participate freely in any intimacy? What other factors are there, such as frequent urinary-tract infections, which may suggest sexual activity?

If there is sexual intimacy that requires lubrication, is it consensual and a natural part of this couple's relationship? How might the team open a discussion with Pauline, Mr Evans and themselves, which explores how they might support this aspect of their changing relationship while ensuring themselves that Pauline is happy to participate, and this is not an instance of abuse? As we can see, this is a complex situation, with part of the dilemma being the informing of staff in relation to their concerns and issues. One way forward could be a conversation with Mr Evans about Pauline's frequent urine infections as a way of opening the dialogue. If willing, Mr Evans, Pauline and the team could go on to talk about ways to manage the intimacy in their relationship to reduce infections and take account of consent and the imminent move to a care home permanently.

In situations such as this, older people do wish for independence, which is accompanied by information, advice and advocacy; in short, they wish to be listened to and spoken to (Denning, 2005).

Recognising abuse

Abuse can occur anywhere with any older person; there is no social class barrier (Action on Elder Abuse, 2004; Manthorpe, 2005). Some key areas of practice are for nurses:

- to be watchful of changes in the older person's behaviour, appearance, habits or morale;
- to be aware of hints of abuse or neglect;
- to talk to the older persons to see if they are afraid or want a confident or support;
- to keep the person's safety in focus;
- to preserve evidence and keep accurate records, perhaps by keeping body maps to indicate the size, colour and location of any injury in addition to good note keeping;
- to share any concerns with team members or their managers, or, if nothing is done, to a higher level, i.e. whistle blowing;
- to seek support for themselves through supervision as they address abuse.

Conclusions

By acting on our duty of care to older people, we can build a toolbox of techniques and evidence-based intervention to make the management of dilemmas

Box 7.1   Key skills for dealing with mental-health dilemmas

- The ability to assess the risks by using key questions, such as those offered here.
- The ability to be clear in checking out your own assumptions.
- The ability to constantly check out consent with the older person.
- The planning of interventions as a team which involves the older person.
- Remembering the therapeutic approaches and trying them out, 24-hour reality orientation, a biographical approach and validation to start.
- Using intuition and skill to keep the communication going with the older person using other therapeutic approaches as needed.
- Being systematic if using restraint, review and reflect on its impact and return to therapeutic approaches as soon as the risk has passed.
- The ability to act when abuse is suspected or recognised.
- Keeping your toolbox of skills and expertise 'live' and remaining open to learning new skills.

in mental health care easier to navigate. By keeping focused on the voices of older people and their agendas, we can look behind the behaviour to the core reasons for difficulties and respond appropriately. When we check out our own assumptions as practitioners, we can build our skills and confidence, and assure ourselves that we identify the right times for restraint to be used and undertake it with skill and care in partnership with older people.

Box 7.1 shows key skills for dealing with mental health dilemmas.

References

2006 Commission for Healthcare Audit and Inspection (2006) *Living Well in Later Life. A Service Review of the Progress Made Against the National Service Framework for Older People.* London, CHAI.

Action on Elder Abuse (2004) *Hidden Voices. Older People's Experience of Abuse.* London, Help the Aged.

Action on Elder Abuse (2006) *What is elder abuse?* http://www.elderabuse.org.uk

Association of Directors of Social Services (2005) *Safeguarding Adults – Everyone's Business. A National Framework of Standards for Good Practice and Outcomes in Adult Protection Work.* London, Association of Directors of Social Services.

Crump, A. (1998) Disease or distress an exploration of mental health and age. In: *Caring for Older People, Developing Specialist Practice* (J. Marr and B. Kershaw, eds). Bristol, UK, Arnold, pp. 165–189.

Denning, A. (2005) *Information, Advice and Advocacy for Older People, Defining and Developing Services.* York, UK, Joseph Rowntree Foundation.

Department of Health (2000) *No Secrets: Guidance on Developing and Implementing Multi-Agency Policies and Procedures to Protect Vulnerable Adults from Abuse.* London, Department of Health.

Department of Health (2001) *12 Key Points on Consent. The Law in England.* London, Department of Health.

Department of Health (2006) *Protection of Vulnerable Adults (POVA) audit.* http://www.dh.gov.uk/PublicationsAndStatistics

Duff, L., Gray, R. and Bristow, F. (1996) The use of control and restraint techniques in acute psychiatric units. *Psychiatric Care* **3** (6): 230–234.

Feil, N. (2002) *The Validation Breakthrough; Simple Techniques for Communicating with People with Alzheimer's-Type-Dementia.* Baltimore, MD, Health Professionals Press.

Levenson. R. (1998) *Drugs and Dementia, a Guide to Good Practice in the Use of Neuroleptic Drugs in Care Homes for Older People.* London, Age Concern.

McCormack, B. (2005) Underpinning values. In: *Older People: Assessment for Health and Social Care* (H. Heath and R. Watson, eds). London, Age Concern, pp. 44–52.

Manthorpe J (2005) Preventing and responding to elder abuse. In: *Older People: Assessment for Health and Social Care* (H. Heath and R. Watson, eds). London, Age Concern, pp. 263–270.

Melia, K. (2004) *Health Care Ethics.* London, Sage.

Nursing and Midwifery Council (2004) *Code of Professional Conduct.* London, Nursing and Midwifery Council.

Phair L (1999) Mental health. In: *Healthy Ageing Nursing Older People* (H. Heath and I. Schofield, eds). London, Mosby, pp. 407–433.

Royal College of Nursing (2004) *Restraint Revisited: Rights, Risks and Responsibilities; Guidance for Nurses Working with Older People.* London, Royal College of Nursing.

Taylor, H. (2005) *Assessing the Nursing and Care Needs of Older Adults, a Patient Centred Approach.* Oxford, Radcliffe, pp. 39–47.

Watson R (2005) Restraint. In: *Older People: Assessment for Health and Social Care* (H. Heath and R. Watson, eds). London, Age Concern, pp. 202–210.

Chapter 8
Assessing Older People with Mental Health Issues

Henry Minardi

Introduction

While discussing the assessment of clients' mental health needs, a consultant geriatrician said in jest, 'You can usually tell if someone is schizophrenic or demented because their toenails and fingernails are dirty, and they need a bath'. It would be nice if assessments were so simple yet accurate! Each assessment is an evolving, incremental gathering and processing of information relevant to the client's situation/needs (see Case Study 8.1).

Case study 8.1

You have been asked by the GP of an 82-year-old man, Albert, through your Community Assessment Team (CAT), to assess his mental-health. The limited information on the SAP referral form was that his wife asked the GP to see him because he was 'acting strangely'. It also states he had been treated for depression 20 years ago after having been made redundant. You ring the doorbell. His wife answers; you introduce yourself and state the reason for your call. She invites you in.

As you enter the house and follow her to the living room where her husband is sitting, it is likely that you are scanning the environment of, Albert and his wife. This scan, however, involves not only vision but also hearing, smell and touch. You have an awareness of how you are feeling as you approach Albert. What you are doing is making a preliminary assessment which helps you get a sense of the environment and people in it. In starting to talk with Albert and his wife, contact is established, and you begin forming an impression of prevailing social, psychological, physical and environmental issues. You are also likely to be assessing any risks, physical or emotional, to Albert and his wife, and yourself. Much of this material is processed through an 'internal dialogue', which gives you some tentative answers and helps you decide how best to open or sustain the assessment.

The above exemplifies the potential complexity of assessment. This chapter will examine what is involved in undertaking an assessment of client/family needs. Although this book is about mental health nursing, to restrict assessment to just the psychological domain of the older person's life would miss other significant and interdependent dimensions of the whole picture. This will be examined through a discussion of the Single Assessment Process (SAP) (Department of Health, 2001)

An important aspect of an effective assessment is the development of a good therapeutic relationship (Moriarty, 2005). This involves being able to gain the client's trust while not colluding with any distorted thinking. To develop a healthy working relationship with clients, it is necessary to use appropriate interventions in a timely way that requires a fluid use of verbal and non-verbal communication skills as well as active listening (Minardi and Riley, 1997).

The final section of this chapter will identify what a mental health assessment for older adults can contain, including a choice of interview structures and standardised assessment tools to support or refute information obtained during the interview. This chapter will provide a general grounding for assessing more specific mental health issues developed in later chapters of the book.

Assessment revisited

Assessment is an integral component of good nursing care as previously discussed extensively (e.g. Yurick et al., 1989; Ritter and Watkins, 1997; Gamble and Brennan, 2000; Draper and Melding, 2001; Heath and Watson, 2005; Taylor, 2005). The above authors have also identified that assessment provides an important beginning to working collaboratively with clients and their carers. However, rather than a single event, it is a continuous process lasting as long as there is contact with a client, their informal and formal carers. Within this process, it is expected that there will be an exploration of client/carer needs in all domains of care: physical, psychological and spiritual. It is necessary not only to consider all of these elements of the individual separately, but also to consider their relationship.

Hayes and Minardi (2005, p. 191) suggest that an assessment should follow the general principles of a person-centred approach, in order to:

- understand the person's strengths and ability to function rather than just focusing on their impairments;
- distinguish between normal and abnormal ageing in the person being assessed;
- screen for possible mental health issues and take appropriate action;
- consider physical health issues, medication and their possible influence on the person's mental health;
- trigger a plan of care, including risk management and appropriate onward referral if required for further assessment, investigations, treatment and care.

With these principles in mind, the assessment can be held in formal or informal environments, using structured, semi-structured or unstructured interview techniques with or without the use of validated assessment tools such as the geriatric depression scale (GDS) (Yesavage et al., 1983). These interview formats will be discussed in more detail later in the chapter.

Although the general principles identified above could be applied to assessing people in all age groups, particular considerations apply when working with older adults. 'Older Adult' is arbitrarily defined as people who are 65 or more years old. This has been outlined in the National Service Framework (NSF) for Older People (Department of Health, 2001), Standard Two, Person Centred Care, Single Assessment Process. Below is a rationale and discussion of the use of SAP when assessing older adults.

The Single Assessment Process

The SAP was introduced and developed in NHS health care as a result of the NSF for Older People (Department of Health, 2001), Standard Two, Person Centred Care. This was initiated because 'Assessments are often duplicated with no coherent approach across health and social care service' (Department of Health, 2001, p. 24). This is, however, not to ignore the complexity of health-care needs of older people (Department of Health, 2000), but to ensure that unnecessary repetition of the same information given by them, such as date of birth, marital status, family, etc. to one agency/profession is not asked again by another agency/profession during an assessment.

SAP has now been firmly established as a national direction for assessing older adults, and detailed guidance on its implementation has been published (Department of Health, 2002a). It is, however, a complex system because of the need for various agencies to share information about the client. As a result, its implementation in different parts of the UK is at various stages. The process identified has been to establish different types of assessment (Box 8.1), from basic to complex, covering a number of domains (Box 8.2). It importantly joins the strands of health and social care together so that the older person's needs are viewed systemically, not in isolation, thus ensuring that mental health practitioners explore all other dimensions of the older adult's life. It also encour-

Box 8.1   The four types of assessment in SAP

Assessment	Purpose
Contact	To establish basic information about the individual such as date of birth, next of kin, GP, living accommodation, plus needs which are met by specific agencies such as district nurses or social services.
Overview	A rounded assessment which addresses social, health and environmental domains within the older adult's life (see below).
Specialist	To explore, in more detail, specific areas of need which were identified in the contact and overview assessments and undertaken by professionals who have an expertise in that area.
Comprehensive	To collate information obtained from the other assessments undertaken, especially when needs are complex, intensive or prolonged. This will provide a comprehensive summary to help decision-making in the provision of health and social care.

Tabulated from information in Department of Health (2002a). *The Single Assessment Process: Guidance for Local Implementation.* London, HMSO.

Box 8.2   SAP assessment domains and sub-domains

User's perspective
- Problems and issues in the user's own words
- User's expectations and motivation

Clinical background
- History of medical problems
- History of falls
- Medication use

Disease prevention
- History of blood-pressure monitoring
- Nutrition
- Vaccination history
- Drinking and smoking history
- Exercise pattern
- History of cervical and breast screening

Personal care and physical well-being
- Personal hygiene, including washing, bathing, toileting and grooming
- Dressing
- Pain
- Oral health
- Foot care
- Tissue viability
- Mobility
- Continence
- Sleeping patterns

Senses
- Sight
- Hearing
- Communication

Mental health
- Cognition including dementia
- Mental health including depression

Relationships
- Social contacts, relationships and involvement
- Caring arrangements

Safety
- Abuse or neglect
- Other aspects of personal safety
- Public safety

Immediate environment and resources
- Care of the home
- Accommodation
- Finances
- Access to local facilities and services

Department of Health (2001) *National Service Framework for Older People*. London, HMSO, p. 32.

ages an examination of what possible links there may be between these and the individual's current presentation.

Although there are a number of Department of Health approved assessment formats that can be used for an overview assessment (Taylor, 2005), it is recognised that in mental health, the interviews and tools already in use are specialised, usually having been validity-, reliability-, specificity- and sensitivity-tested (Department of Health, 2002a). Thus, assessing the mental health need of older adults will continue to be led by mental health professionals, but have the advantage of supporting information from the contact and overview assessments. It is important to note that initially the Department of Health neglected to include the Care Programme Approach (CPA) assessment and documentation as part of SAP. This was quickly rectified when the Department of Health recognised that important aspects of CPA will still need to apply to older individuals with severe and enduring mental health problems but also '… individual older people with depression, dementia and other mental health problems, of sufficient complexity and severity for specialist mental health services to be involved …' (p. 3, Department of Health, 2002b).

The SAP, therefore, ensures that a detailed initial assessment is undertaken which can identify a need for specialist services, such as mental health. Further developments to assessment are in progress to place assessment and care closer to home, i.e. in the community, with the development of a 'Common Assessment Framework' (Department of Health 2006), to further reduce duplication and integrate health and social care. This has been reinforced by the Parliamentary Under Secretary of State for Care Services, who said, 'There will be a specialist mental service for older adults, with a particular emphasis on community mental health teams and memory clinics', and a common assessment framework will be developed over the next 2 years to provide more effective care for those with complex needs (Byrne, 2006).

Assessment, however, is a process with a beginning, middle and end. It may be just a 'one-off' assessment, as can happen with mental health liaison care in a general hospital or continuous for the years of contact between clients and professionals such as with long-term community mental health care. In either situation, it is necessary to develop a sound working relationship. The stronger this relationship has developed, the more likely that effective initial and ongoing assessments can be made. Its strength is not measured in time spent with the client but the quality of that time. It requires an ability to 'be with' the client, reflect during and after the contact, and contribute to the identification of immediate and ongoing mental health needs. To be therapeutic, the foundation of this relationship needs to be established and nurtured.

Therapeutic relationship development

Returning to the vignette above where you are sent a referral by Albert's GP to visit him, it is here, not – inside his house, that your assessment begins.

You read the referral details, and a number of questions arise. What does he look like? What does 'acting strangely' mean? What is the relationship between him and his wife like? What was his past like, and how does his previous depression fit into the present? Many more questions may arise. It is how you manage these questions that will influence your initial interactions, the consequences of which can make the assessment process easy or difficult. This is also where the therapeutic relationship with clients and carers begins, facilitating the initial and ongoing assessments.

The importance of developing a good working relationship – or alliance – with clients and carers cannot be overemphasised. Timely and skilled communications – non-verbal, verbal and active listening – are key components (Minardi and Riley, 1997). Examining each phase separately will provide a sound base for their necessary amalgamation.

One way of thinking about the development of a therapeutic relationship is to consider that it is a process in which it begins, develops, is reflected upon, is reformulated and either ends or is fed back into future interactions with the client. Thinking in terms of phase development implies that each part has some level of impact on the other. Minardi and Hayes (2005) have formulated these phases as interconnecting and having a pre-interaction, interaction and post-interaction function. (Fig 8.1; Box 8.3)

The *pre-interaction phase* begins when a referral letter is received, there is knowledge of an admission or the client/carers are seen entering the emergency interview room. In this model, influences on the total encounter start before any 'face to face' meeting ever takes place (or 'voice to voice' in telephone contacts). A sequence of anticipatory questions or just one statement is formulated before the interview starts, e.g. 'Tell me about yourself'. What also tends to happen is that anticipatory assumptions are made about the encounter, using the scant information provided in the referral letter. At times, it can take a great deal of conscious work to reduce negative influences of these assumptions. This is where regular clinical supervision can help separate what the client actually may be like from the assumptions you have made. It is also at this point that the flow of the client's/carer's verbal and non-verbal discourse can determine how the interaction phase will develop.

The *interaction phase* is divided into three sections: Beginning, Middle or Working and End (Fig. 8.1; Box 8.3). In the beginning section, all of those directly involved in the interaction – clients, carers, professionals – begin to assess each other. This is undertaken by each person in the context of assumptions they have made about each other prior to meeting and their particular way of viewing the world. As a result of these assessments, questions may emerge such as: What relationships may develop? How much trust will there be? What to disclose? What communication techniques are best to use? and Will the interaction continue beyond this encounter? By using communication skills that are exploratory and supportive but not collusive, asking appropriately formulated open and closed questions, active and attentive listening and clarifying any perplexing responses, nurses are more likely to engender a good working relationship (Minardi and Riley, 1997).

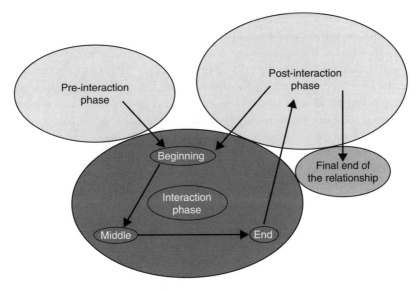

Fig. 8.1 Phases of therapeutic relationship development. Adapted from Minardi, H. and Hayes, N (2005). Communication. In: *Older People: Assessment for Health and Social Care* (Heath, H. and Watson, R., eds) London, Age Concern, pp. 211–228. Used with permission.

Box 8. 3 Phases of therapeutic relationship development

1. *Pre-interaction phase*
    a. Anticipation of the contact and interactions
    b. Assumptions about the person and relationships
    c. Preoccupation with the request for contact
    d. Purpose of the interaction
 	
2. *Interaction phase*
    a. Beginning
       i. The relationship fluctuates between distant and close
      ii. Higher proportion of general rather than specific statements/questions, which helps establish the relationship development
     iii. Balance between general and specific discussion
    b. Middle (working)
       i. Therapeutic work
    c. Ending
       i. Ending the contact/relationship
 	
3. *Post-interaction phase*
    a. Reflection on the interaction which took place and its relationship to the whole encounter
    b. Further development of present relationship with client/carers/professionals
    c. Maintenance of the future relationship with present client/carers
 	
It is important to acknowledge that the phases are relevant to all individuals - clients, carers, and professionals – involved in the interactions

Adapted from Minardi, H. and Hayes, N. (2005), Communication. In: *Older People: Assessment for Health and Social Care* (H. Heath and R. Watson eds). London, Age Concern. pp. 211–228. Used with permission.

The aim is to move the interaction into the middle (working) section of the interaction phase which will begin to focus more on the purpose of the assessment, whether it is a first assessment or part of a long-term therapeutic relationship where assessment is continuous. Forchuk et al. (1998) found that listening and consistency were important for the relationship to develop into a working one. Thus, in the middle section of the interaction phase, the client and/or carer is encouraged to share more in-depth material relevant to the purpose of their contact with the nurse. It can offer insights to help appreciate client/carer needs and wishes. It will also offer insights into the strengths clients and carers have, but as yet do not recognise, to help them manage the difficulties they are experiencing. Interventions during this section can also challenge any distortions in thinking or beliefs the client may hold with a view to working on possible change. The ending stage of this phase may signify a temporary break until the next encounter or permanent ending, depending upon the purpose of the relationship. It is also important to recognise that the process involved in the interaction phase is continuous throughout each routine encounter between the client and nurse.

The *post-interaction phase* of relationship development occurs when contact between the nurse and client ends. This may be prior to the next meeting, which could be within a few minutes or the next day/week. It would also occur when there are no further meetings such as in some liaison mental health assessments when a 'one-off' mental health nursing assessment is required. During this phase, what Schön (1983) describes as 'reflection on practice' takes place to examine the interaction that has just occurred, and see what communication techniques can be altered/added for subsequent or new encounters. Also, depending on the emotional content of the interaction, this reflective process may recur with the practitioner until the next encounter with the client. It is important that regular clinical supervision is in place, so the thinking which underpins this interaction does not interfere in other aspects of care the nurse needs to undertake with this or another client.

The working relationship needs to be enclosed in an envelope of psychological safety for sufficient trust to develop (Minardi and Hayes, 2003). The core conditions of genuineness, acceptance and accurate empathy are key components of such a matrix. It is through this safe environment that the client will recognise that they are being listened to and understood, important elements of an accurate assessment.

Accurate and active listening is central to undertaking an assessment of clients' mental health needs (Minardi and Riley, 1997). A large proportion of nursing time in clinical practice revolves around requests, entreaties, concerns, orders and advice. It is not surprising that at times, we defend against this onslaught by attending selectively to clients. However, when working with people, be they colleagues or clients, it is important for them to be able to recognise that they are being listened to with attention and understanding.

Effective listening is an active process involving attending to communication (both verbal and non-verbal), processing and interpreting its meaning and conveying your understanding to the client – verbally and non-verbally. The listener's non-verbal communication such as posture, movements, gestures, gaze and overall appearance will have a key role in indicating to the client that they are being listened to and valued. Conversely, nurses may prevent clients from feeling that they are being listened to and understood by interrupting, allowing or responding to interruptions by others, appearing preoccupied, being over-informative, and inappropriately directive. In order to recognise such behaviours in ourselves, we need to be aware of our responses. In an interesting study by Kemper et al. (1998), young participants unconsciously used a type of speech they termed 'elderspeak' – with older adults characterised as speaking slowly, using uncomplicated grammatical structure, repetition and shorter sentences – i.e. an assumption of cognitive impairment when there is none. Thus, by being aware of the way you communicate with a client and/or carer, the assessment you make is less likely to be biased by assumptions which may be prejudicial.

There is, however, one caveat to be considered. Dryden and Feltham (1994) found that, no matter how skilled a professional is at communicating, other factors such as age, gender, race, personality differences, etc. can be barriers to conducting a constructive assessment. It must be recognised that such barriers can originate from the client or nurse. It is important that these problem areas be recognised and used by nurses to try to overcome, at least partially, their impact on the assessment.

Structure of mental health assessments

The importance of developing a good working relationship with the older adult when assessing their mental health cannot be over-emphasised. Similarly, having a good working knowledge of normal ageing processes, as discussed in Chapters 1, 2 and 3, is of equal importance. The complexity of health and social issues affecting an older adult should not automatically be attributed to a mental health problem. In order to avoid inappropriate attributions, some framework needs to be applied to the assessment.

As stated earlier in this paper, an assessment can be structured, semistructured or unstructured. It can also use validated measurement tools, such as a screening test, to support findings from the interview or to mark progress. Although the purpose of a mental health assessment is to identify client needs, to focus only on mental health issues would miss factors that can strongly influence an older person's mental health. Thus, to approach assessment as being systemic, i.e., exploring systems internal (e.g., anatomical, functional, psychological) and external (e.g. familial, social, economic) to the individual, is necessary as each has an impact upon the other.

It has been identified that the NSF for Older People contains nine domains, each with a number of sub-domains, to make up an overview assessment (Box 8.2). This, however, does not have enough depth or breadth to effectively undertake mental health assessments. Also, because of multiple issues which a client may present, it only provides 'starter' information which must be followed-up during subsequent meetings. The mental health assessment needs to be broad enough to encompass external systems and deep enough to explore internal systems with the ultimate goal of combining the outcomes to provide the basis of a holistic care plan. The complexity of such an assessment would be difficult to complete in a single interview, though in some branches of mental health nursing, this may be all that is available such as in liaison mental health care. Within the spectrum of a single interview to ongoing contact, it is useful to explore what needs to be assessed and where the priorities lie.

What will be assessed?

When a referral is made to assess someone in their own home, someone in a registered care home or pending admission to a mental health unit in hospital, you will have received some information about the person. Initially, you try to understand the information you have received and then begin to formulate the areas you will explore with the client – and possibly carers – deciding where the priorities might lie but also recognising that once you are face to face, these priorities might change. However, the question of risk must be present, regardless of what information you have received about the person.

Risk assessment is an activity which is regularly undertaken in ordinary life (Manthorpe, 2005). We assess the probability of an outcome as a result of an action we take. For example, when crossing a busy road, we assess when and where it is best for us to cross. With an older adult, this assessment becomes more complex because vision, hearing and mobility may be poor, all factors which increase risk. With older adults risk is not just about deliberate self-harm or harm to others; it can relate to what others may do to them, i.e. elder abuse. Other factors, though still pertaining to younger adults, are more likely to occur with older people such as self-neglect, wandering as a result of delirium or dementia or falls. Thus, risk assessment is more complex and best undertaken, when possible, through multi-disciplinary working (Ritter and Watkins, 1997). In this way, assessing risk not only provides mutual support for findings of the assessment but also affords discussion of appropriate risk-taking to enhance the quality of a client's life. This acknowledges that assessment of risk is formulated by good clinical judgement, not just a validated risk-assessment tool (Ryrie, 2000).

All health-care trusts will have risk-assessment instruments. With older adults, risk assessment has become part of the SAP. Generally, these tools are similar and include items such as dangerous use of domestic appliances, risk of self-harm, risk of severe self-neglect, risk of falling, risk of elder abuse, risk related to physical condition and risk from polypharmacy or non-compliance with treatment. However, there are no instruments which can predict with a high degree of accuracy which risks are more likely to manifest (Ryrie, 2000). Thus, assessment of risk is usually undertaken during the process of the first

Box 8.4   Assessment interview topics

Overview (This is to obtain a whole view of the client and their life)
- Present physical and mental health status
- Presenting complaint and its history
- Medical and psychiatric history
- Personal, family and social history
- Present habits, routines and coping strategies
- Present social situation, including social functioning and support, finances and housing
- Meaningful daily activities
- Quality of life
- Medicines used and their effect

Present mental health status (This is to focus specifically on their mental-health)
- Present and past personality features
- Behaviour and presentation
- Speech abnormalities
- Mood disturbances
- Distortions in thinking
- Abnormal perceptions
- Cognition
- Insight into presenting mental health issues
- Use of alcohol, non-prescribed drugs (including analgesia) and tobacco

---

Box 8.5   Assessing suicide risk

- Do you ever feel life is not worth living?
- Do you have a sense of hopelessness?
- Do you find that it is getting more difficult to think about living as days go on?
- Have you ever thought about doing something about it?
- Have you thought about harming yourself?
- Do you think you would try to kill yourself?
- Are you able to stop yourself from thinking about harming yourself?
- If not, what would stop you from trying to commit suicide?
- Have you attempted suicide in the past?
- What method might you use to kill yourself?
- Do you know how you might do this?
- How likely is it that you might carry out this plan?
- If your first method of harming yourself is not available, what other ways might you try?
- What else would you like to say about trying to kill yourself?

Depending upon the response you get and whether you feel it is a true reflection of the client's thoughts, you may skip some of these questions.

---

assessment (Box 8.4), though a more detailed risk assessment of deliberate self harm (DSF) may be warranted after this initial assessment (Box 8.5).

A mental health assessment can be broadly divided into Specialist Overview and Present Mental Health Status (Box 8.4). With older adults, the domains of physical health and medication are important inclusions in an assessment of their mental health. This is because there is more likely to be polypharmacy and physical ill health with older adults than with younger adults. For example, it is common to find older people on medication known to have depression as a side effect, e.g. drugs for cardiac problems or gastric reflux. In Parkinson's disease (PD), which most commonly occurs in adults over the age of 55, the medication used can cause psychotic symptoms such as visual hallucinations (Turjanski and Lloyd, 2005). However, PD itself can be a cause of psychotic symptoms (Calne, 2005). Also, it is well documented that physical ill health can be a cause of depression in older adults (Braam et al., 2005).

Therefore, both physical and mental health must be assessed. However, just as important is the individual's social world, as this can also contribute to the mental health of older adults. For example, a reduction in perceived social support can contribute to depression (Prince et al., 1997).

How will it be assessed?

An assessment can be undertaken in a formal or informal environment, with a rigid or loose structure and/or using a valid assessment tool. Table 8.1 provides a matrix identifying the types of structure and environment which may be used when assessing someone's mental health needs. However, note that in the matrix, none of the cells are dedicated solely to an assessment tool. This is because such an instrument can only provide a limited amount of information relating to the focus of that tool, such as using the Mania Rating Scale (Bech et al., 1978) to quantify the severity of a person's manic state or the Mini Mental State Examination (Folstein et al., 1975) to identify the level of cognitive deficit present in a client. Therefore, it is only with the concomitant information provided by an interview that a broader understanding of the client's needs may be elicited.

In the assessment matrix, there are 12 possible permutations for undertaking an assessment (Table 8.1). Options 1A and B and 2A and B are likely to be used more by those practitioners who are new to the work of assessing clients' mental health needs. In this circumstance, following rules is important for some stability when learning new practice (Benner, 1984). Options 5A and B and 6A and B are likely to be undertaken by a very skilled practitioner who is time-limited and clear about what issue needs assessing. Options 3A and B and 4A and B are where the majority of assessments are likely to fall. Here, the assessment areas identified in Boxes 8.2, 8.4 and 8.5 will be addressed, though there is also freedom to follow a theme which the client wants to focus upon or the assessor recognises as being fundamental to helping the client meet a need.

Using a semi-structured interview format allows a free flow of information between the client – and/or carer – and practitioner, ensuring that appropriate themes are addressed. Such a format can follow the interaction direction of the client while still ensuring that there is discussion of client needs which they may not realise exist. In order to optimise this interview style, the nurse must keep 'in mind' what the client has disclosed. Thus, when using format 3B, semi-structured/informal, a second assessment to clarify an issue that was

Table 8.1 Assessment interview matrix

Assessment structure	Environment setting	
	(a) Formal environment	(b) Informal environment
Option 1 Structured without Assessment Tool	E.g. Present Mental Health Status * topic areas covered in strict order, in an office or specifically designated interview room	E.g. Present Mental Health Status * topic areas covered in strict order, in the client's home, in a ward lounge, in a surgery waiting room
Option 2 Structured with Assessment Tool	E.g. Present Mental Health Status * topic areas covered in strict order, in an office or specifically designated interview room using a specific instrument(s), e.g. BASDEC**	E.g. Present Mental Health Status * topic areas covered in strict order, in the client's home, in a ward lounge, in a surgery waiting room using a specific instrument(s), e.g. the BASDEC**
Option 3 Semi-structured without Assessment Tool	E.g. Present Mental Health Status * with all of the exam areas covered but not in a specific order, in an office or specifically designated interview room	E.g. Present Mental Health Status * with all of the exam areas covered but not in a specific order, in the client's home, in a ward lounge or in a surgery waiting room
Option 4 Semi-structured with Assessment Tool	E.g. Present Mental Health Status * with all of the exam areas covered but not in a specific order, in an office or specifically designated interview room using a specific instrument(s), e.g. BASDEC**	E.g. Present Mental Health Status * with all of the exam areas covered but not in a specific order, in the client's home, in a ward lounge or in a surgery waiting room using a specific instrument(s), e.g. the BASDEC**
Option 5 Unstructured without Assessment Tool	E.g. interviewing the client in an office or designated interview room randomly gaining information, and not covering all mental-state topics, about psychiatric problems the client may be experiencing	E.g. interviewing the client in their home, in a ward lounge, in a surgery waiting room randomly gaining information, and not covering all mental-state topics, about psychiatric problems the client may be experiencing
Option 6 Unstructured with Assessment Tool	E.g. interviewing the client in an office or designated interview room randomly gaining information, and not covering all mental-state topics, about psychiatric problems the client may be experiencing using an assessment tool specific to the area under discussion, e.g. BASDEC**	E.g. interviewing the client in their home, in a ward lounge or in a surgery waiting room randomly gaining information, and not covering all mental-state topics, about psychiatric problems the client may be experiencing using an assessment tool specific to the area under discussion, e.g. BASDEC**.

*See Box 8.4 - Present Mental Health Status.

Adshead, F., Day, C.D. and Pitt, B. (1992). BASDEC (Brief Assessment Schedule Depression Cards): a novel screening instrument for depression in elderly medical inpatients. *British Medical Journal* **305, 397.

previously unclear can be accomplished at the same time as discussing daily activities. This format is likely to be more satisfactory for the practitioner and client because, whether in a formal or informal setting, it becomes more conversational and allows the client to tell their 'story', which helps the practitioner gain some insight into the person, not just their presenting problems (Wells 2005). Using a semi-structured format helps in the development of rapport between the client and nurse, helps build the psychologically safe atmosphere identified earlier in this chapter and provides some insight into the clients living patterns and coping behaviours (Fox and Conroy, 2000).

The flexibility of a semi-structured interview when assessing can facilitate the introduction of psychometric tests. These, however, are best used to support – or refute – clinical evidence obtained through interview rather than diagnostically. They can also be used more than once with a client as part of a reassessment and progress marker.

Common tests used are the Geriatric Depression Scale (GDS; Yesavage et al., 1983) and the Mini-Mental State (MMSE; Folstein et al., 1975). Other tests, such as the Mania Rating Scale (MRS; Bech et al., 1978) to quantify the severity of mania, or the Brief Psychiatric Rating Scale (BPRS; Overall and Gorham, 1962) and Geriatric Mental State Schedule (GMSS; Copeland et al., 1976) for a global assessment of psychopathology can also be used as an adjunct to an interview. A note of caution, however, needs to be made when using psychometric tests. Deviation from their original format and content would bring their validity and reliability into question. Also, some populations may be disadvantaged by the tests, e.g., people with a low level of education can perform less well on the MMSE (Anthony et al., 1982). A very helpful reference source is the book by Burns et al. (1999) of over 150 psychometric tests designed for use with older adults.

What will be done with the assessment?

The assessment becomes part of care planning with the client. This care planning, when skilfully carried out, will use the information gathered from assessments, using positive coping strategies of clients and trying, where possible, to help clients recognise and alter distorted strategies which may have had a deleterious effect on their mental health. Its success will be assisted by involving the client, and carer when appropriate, in all assessments, care planning and evaluation. Just as with each phase of assessment and relationship development, using the skilled communication and the assessment themes identified in this chapter will help ensure that the therapeutic contact with clients and carers, regardless of the environment, will result in the most appropriate care for that client.

Conclusion

This chapter has focused on the assessment process of older adults with suspected mental health needs. The assessment of specific areas of mental health will be addressed elsewhere. The concept of assessment itself has been revisited. Its complexity with older adults has been highlighted because this population is more likely to be affected by *physical health issues*: polypharmacy, frequent infections, decreased mobility; *social issues*: decreased independence, deaths, financial concerns, housing; and *psychological issues*: multiple personal and relationship losses, fears and loneliness.

A collaborative therapeutic relationship needs to be formed in order for an assessment to be truly genuine and of benefit to the client. Phases of relationship development and associated communication, have been described. This model can help the nurse/practitioner keep the client 'in mind' so they can benefit from the nurses reflection both 'on' and 'in' practice.

The structure and content of assessment were considered, with or without a psychometric instrument. Which structure is used, and how it is used, depends upon the client's presenting emotional state, the practitioner's experience, time available and/or themes requiring further assessment.

The overarching messages are:

- Assessment is not a 'single entity' (unless circumstances makes this appropriate, e.g. a mental capacity assessment in liaison mental health care) but a series of encounters to help nurses understand the client as a whole person with strengths, weaknesses, loves and losses.
- Older adults do not want multiple repetitions of information they give, hence the single assessment process where basic information is asked only once.
- One of the most important aspects of a good assessment is the building of a therapeutic relationship where collaborative working occurs and communication flows easily and safely between the nurse and client (and carers).
- Finally, the assessment environment and structure are such that it allows the client to experience the assessment/reassessment as a process in which they feel valued, listened to and safe.

References

Adshead, F., Day, C.D. and Pitt, B. (1992). BASDEC (Brief Assessment Schedule Depression Cards): a novel screening instrument for depression in elderly medical inpatients. *British Medical Journal* **305**, 397.

Anthony, J.C., LeResche, L., Niaz, U., Von Korff, M.R. and Folstein, M.F. (1982). Limits of the 'Mini-Mental State' as a screening test for dementia and delirium among hospital Patients. *Psychological Medicine* **12**, 397–408.

Bech, P., Rafaelsen, O.J., Kramp, P. and Bolwig, T.G. (1978). The Mania Rating Scale: scale construction and inter-observer agreement. *Neuropharmacology* **17**, 430–431.

Benner, P.E. (1984). *From Novice to Expert: Excellence and Power in Clinical Nursing Practice.* Menlo Park, CA, Addison-Wesley.

Braam, A.W., Prince, M.J., Beekman, A.T., et al. (2005). Physical health and depressive symptoms in older Europeans: Results from EURODEP. *British Journal of Psychiatry* **187**, 35–42.

Burns, A., Lawlor, B. and Craig, S. (1999). *Assessment Scales in Old Age Psychiatry.* London, Martin Dunitz.

Byrne, L. (2006). Speech by Liam Byrne MP, Parliamentary Under Secretary of State for Care Services, 19 April 2006, Care and Health Seminar, CBI Conference Centre.

Calne, S. (2005). Late-stage Parkinson's disease for the rehabilitation specialist: a nursing perspective. *Topics in Geriatric Rehabilitation* **21** (3), 233–246.

Copeland, J.R.M., Kelleher, M.J., Kellett, J.M., Gourlay, A.J., Gurland, B.J., Fleiss, J.L. and Sharpe, L. (1976). A semi-structured clinical interview for the assessment of diagnosis and mental state in the elderly: The Geriatric Mental State Schedule: I. Development and reliability. *Psychological Medicine* **6**, 439–449.

Department of Health (2000) *The NHS Plan.* London, HMSO.

Department of Health (2001) *National Service Framework for Older People.* London, HMSO.

Department of Health (2002a) *The Single Assessment Process: Guidance for Local Implementation.* London, HMSO.

Department of Health (2002b) *Care Management for Older People with Serious Mental Health Problems.* London, HMSO.

Department of Health (2006) *Our Health, Our Care, Our Say: a New Direction for Community Services.* London, HMSO.

Draper, B. and Melding, P. (2001) The Assessment. In: *Geriatric Consultation Liaison Psychiatry* (P. Melding and B. Draper, eds). Oxford, Oxford University Press, pp. 109–139.

Dryden, W. and Feltham, C. (1994) *Developing the Practice of Counselling.* London, Sage.

Folstein, M.F., Folstein, S.E. and McHugh, P.R. (1975) 'Mini-Mental State': A practical method for grading the cognitive state of patients for the clinician. *Journal of Psychiatric Research* **12**, 189–198.

Forchuk, C., Westwell, J., Martin, M.-L., Azzapardi, W.B., Kosterewa-Tolman, D. and Hux, M. (1998) Factors influencing movement of chronic psychiatric patients from the orientation to the working phase of the nurse–client relationship on an inpatient unit. *Perspectives in Psychiatric Care* **34** (1), 36–44.

Fox, J. and Conroy, P. (2000) Assessing client's needs: the semistructured interview. In: *Working with Serious Mental Illness: A Manual for Clinical Practice* (C. Gamble and G. Brennan, eds). Edinburgh, Baillière Tindall, pp. 85–96.

Gamble, C. and Brennan, G. (2000) Assessments: a rationale and glossary of terms. In: *Working with Serious Mental Illness: A Manual for Clinical Practice* (C. Gamble and G. Brennan, eds). Edinburgh, Baillière Tindall, pp. 67–84.

Hayes, N and Minardi, H (2005) Memory and cognition. In: *Older People: Assessment for Health and Social Care* (H. Heath and R. Watson, eds). London, Age Concern, pp. 188–201.

Heath, H. and Watson, R. (Eds) (2005) *Older People: Assessment for Health and Social Care.* London, Age Concern.

Kemper, S., Finter-Urczyk, A., Ferrell, P., Harden, T. and Billington, C. (1998) Using elderspeak with older adults. *Discourse Processes* **25** (1), 55–73.

Manthorpe, J. (2005). Rights and risk. In *Older People: Assessment for Health and Social Care* (H. Heath and R. Watson, eds). London, Age Concern, pp. 229–235.

Minardi, H. and Hayes, N. (2005). Communication. In: *Older People: Assessment for Health and Social Care* (H. Heath and R. Watson, eds). London, Age Concern, pp. 211–228.

Minardi, H. and Hayes, N. (2003) Nursing older people with mental health problems: therapeutic interventions – part 2. *Nursing Older People* **15** (7), 20–24.

Minardi, H.A. and Riley, M.J. (1997) *Communication in Health Care: a Skills-Based Approach.* Oxford: Butterworth-Heinemann.

Moriarty, J. (2005) *Update for SCIE Best Practice Guide on Assessing the Mental Health Needs of Older People.* London, Social Care Workforce Research Unit, Kings College.

Overall, J.E. and Gorham, D.R. (1962) The Brief Psychiatric Rating Scale. *Psychological Reports* **10**, 799–812.

Prince, M.J., Harwood, R.H., Blizard, R.A. and Mann, A.H. (1997) Social support deficits, loneliness and life events as risk factors for depression in old age. The Gospel Oak Project V. *Psychological Medicine* **27**, 323–332.

Ritter, S. and Watkins, M. (1997) Assessment of older people. In: *Mental Health Care for Elderly People* (I.J. Norman and S.J. Redfern, eds). Edinburgh, Churchill Livingstone, pp. 99–130.

Ryrie, I. (2000) Assessing risk. In: *Working with Serious Mental Illness: A Manual for Clinical Practice* (C. Gamble and G. Brennan, eds). Edinburgh: Baillière Tindall, pp. 97–111.

Schön, D.A. (1983) *The Reflective Practitioner: How Professionals Think in Action*. New York, Basic Books.

Taylor, H. (2005) *Assessing the Nursing and Care Needs of Older Adults: A Patient-Centred Approach*. Oxford, Radcliffe.

Turjanski, N. and Lloyd, G.G. (2005) Psychiatric side-effects of medications: recent developments. *Advances in Psychiatric Treatment*, **11**, 58–70.

Wells, D. (2005) Biographical and developmental approaches. In: *Older People: Assessment for Health and Social Care* (H. Heath and R. Watson, eds), pp. 54–63. London, Age Concern.

Yesavage, J.A., Brink, T.L., Rose, T.L., Lum, O., Huang, V., Adey, M. and Leirer, V.O. (1983) Development and validation of a geriatric depression screening scale: A preliminary report. *Journal of Psychiatric Research* **17** (1), 37–49.

Yurick, A.G., Spier, B.E., Robb, S.S. and Ebert, N.J. (1989) *The Aged Person and the Nursing Process*, 3rd edn. Norwalk, CT, Appleton Lange.

Part 3
NEGLECTED ASPECTS

Chapter 9
Culture, Religion and Spirituality

Peter Draper and Wilfred McSherry

Introduction

The National Service Framework (NSF) for Older People (Department of Health 2001b, p. 1) suggests that during the period 1995–2025, the number of people between the ages of 65 and 90 will double. This has important implications for the provision of health and social care, both in terms of the extent of that provision, and for the ways in which the needs of older people are understood. However, it is important that older people are not simply regarded as a needy group occupying the 'debit' side of the social balance sheet, for they (we?) are also a resource whose experience, ways of understanding and knowledge offer a major contribution to society.

Within the last decade, it has increasingly been recognised by researchers and health and social care professionals that the physical and mental health of all people, irrespective of gender, creed, culture, race or ethnicity, are maintained by addressing a number of interrelated dimensions within a holistic approach (Cornah, 2006). The dimensions are described as the physical, psychological, social and spiritual (Department of Health 2001a, b). There has been a shift away from seeing people (especially older people) just as physical beings, and attention is now turning to other fundamental areas of the older persons' life such as relationships, belief systems, cultural, religious and spiritual practices and recreational activities. This chapter begins with a brief exploration of the nature of spirituality before discussing the importance of culture and religion and finally discussing assessment for culturally sensitive care.

Spirituality

The subject of spirituality has received a great deal of attention within the nursing literature. See, for example, Culliford (2002), for a discussion in relation to psychiatry, and Nolan and Crawford (1997), Greasley et al. (2001), Coleman (2006), and Thomas (2006), who relate it to mental health nursing. However, there is still a great deal of uncertainty about what the term 'spirituality' means. Thus, Narayanasamy (2001) considers there to be no authoritative definition of the concept, and McSherry (2006) recognises that there is a diversity of opinion on the topic.

A number of authors offer definitions of spirituality, and it may be helpful to review these. MacKinlay (1998, p. 36) suggests that spirituality is:

'That which lies at the core of each person's being, an essential dimension which brings meaning to life. It is acknowledged that spirituality is not constituted only by religious practices, but must be understood more broadly, as relationship with God, however God or ultimate meaning is perceived by the person, and in relationship with other people.'

In a similar contemporary definition, Confoy (2002, p. 27) argues that in its widest meaning, spirituality not only goes beyond, but also includes, people's beliefs, convictions and patterns of thoughts, their emotions and behaviour in respect to what is ultimate or to God. The ways people relate to each other and to their environment influence the shape their spirituality takes. Their place in society, life circumstances, the rituals and patterns of living, loving and working contribute to their spiritual development (cf. Carr, 1988, p. 203). Spirituality is also shaped by personal, familial and cultural storytelling that tells us who we are and about our place in the world.

Finally, Coleman (2006, p. 113) suggests: '... that spirituality is critical to the essence of our health and to our relationships with others. However defined or classified, it is core to having a meaningful and purposeful existence'.

Against the background of these definitions, our own view is that the concept of spirituality is an attempt to recognise and value the deepest and most fundamental characteristics of human beings: their fears and aspirations; their relationships with one another and with the world; the symbolic and linguistic structures of religious and secular world views through which they create, express and experience meaning; and the ways in which they deal with fear, illness and death and other major life transitions.

It is perhaps inevitable that a concept used to express and explore such a wide range of issues will be the focus of debate and even disagreement; but many contemporary researchers and practitioners also seem to find that the concept of spirituality enables them to explore a range of important issues that might otherwise be neglected. The implication of all this is that there is no simple way to discuss the contribution of spirituality to the mental health of older people; but in this chapter, we hope to bring the concept to bear on a number of relevant issues and perhaps illuminate them from a spiritual perspective.

At a practical level, we suggest that these definitions of spirituality illustrate ways in which the concept of spirituality might usefully be related to the mental health of older people. For example, many older people will experience loss, either of a spouse or partner through bereavement, or of their own health. The experience of loss can constitute an existential challenge; but equally, spiritual resources can offer a way of coping with this change. Golsworthy and Coyle (1999) suggest that religious and spiritual beliefs are an important way in which human beings create a structure of meaning that gives a sense of order and purpose to existence and to death, and in a phenomenological study they explore older people's understanding of loss from a spiritual perspective.

The work of Deborah Dunn (2004) gives an interesting illustration of strategies developed to meet the spiritual needs of persons with dementia in an acute hospital unit. She argues simply that spiritual care means 'care for the whole person ... and what is meaningful in their life' (p. 154) and describes how she uses tools such as narrative gerontology (story telling) and validation therapy (listening with empathy) to achieve outcomes related to family relationships, the expression of grief, the provision of mutual support, building confidence and coping with fear.

The importance of culture

Culture plays an important role in determining behaviour and attitudes, and it is particularly significant in relation to spirituality, religion and mental health. But what is culture? Helman (2001, p. 2) gives the following account:

'... one can see that culture is a set of guidelines (both explicit and implicit) that individuals inherit as members of a particular society and that tells them how to view the world, how to experience it emotionally, and how to behave in it in relation to other people, to supernatural forces or gods, and to the natural environment. It also provides them with a way of transmitting these guidelines to the next generation – by the use of symbols, language, art and ritual. To some extent, culture can be seen as an inherited "lens" through which the individual perceives and understands the world that he inhabits, and learns how to live within it.'

The idea that we inherit and transmit culture has important implications for our understanding of the mental health of older people, as competing cultural perspectives, which may be either implicit or explicit, help to determine how we understand mental health and cope with mental health problems.

The notion of professional culture offers an interesting illustration of the concept. Research shows that new recruits to any profession undergo a period of 'professional socialisation' during which they are exposed to the attitudes, behaviours and values of their professional peer group (see, for example, Melia, 1987, for an account of professional socialisation into nursing). Professional culture may share some of the features of the surrounding culture, but in other respects it may be distinct.

Historically, within the culture of professional nursing, working with older people in 'geriatric' or 'psycho-geriatric' settings was regarded as menial and given a low status. Indeed, both of the authors of this chapter were advised against applying for posts involving work with older people on the basis that this would be detrimental to career development. Negative attitudes towards older people may be transmitted from one generation of nurses to the next through socialisation in the practice setting (Haight et al., 1994; MacKinlay and

Cowan, 2003; McLafferty and Morrison, 2004). This cycle can be broken through education and positive role models within the practice setting.

Culture can also be important in determining how mental health and its attendant problems are understood. Historically, the culture of professional health care has focused upon the disease process, and service provision has been provided according to a biological or medical model of care in which priority is given to correcting biochemical or structural abnormalities (McSherry, 2006). The focus within this model is not on the older person as an 'individual', but on the nature of the disease process (for example, dementia or depression). Although this model is relatively successful in the acute setting, its failures as an organising principle for promoting the well-being of older people have been recognised for many years (see, for example, Baker 1978, Draper 1994). This is why recent policy and strategic developments such as the NSF (Department of Health 2001b) for older people recommend a holistic approach when caring for older people, including spiritual and psychological domains (see Standard Seven, which is devoted to 'Mental health in older people'). The importance of the holistic approach in which psychosocial and spiritual issues are recognised in the context of mental health is also reflected in contemporary professional research (Swinton, 2001; Webb, 2004). Furthermore, the idea of a single multi-agency assessment (Department of Health 2001b) addressing fundamental aspects of the older person signals a paradigm shift from viewing older people as isolated, disconnected individuals, to locating them within a context, involving the family and wider community.

The concept of culture is not restricted to professionals, for arguably, all human beings are brought up in a cultural context and reflect cultural values in their behaviour and attitudes. In the modern world, it is increasingly difficulty to avoid the fact that we share social space with people whose cultural values may be different from our own. In some circumstances, the experience of cultural difference can be liberating as one is exposed to new ways of seeing and understanding the world; but at other times, the experience of cultural difference may lead to mistrust and even hostility.

Against this background, it is particularly important to remember that spirituality is expressed and understood in a cultural context. The work of McSherry (2004) provides an illustrative example. McSherry interviewed patients and professionals to find out what they understood by the term 'spirituality'. He discovered two competing 'discourses' or ways of understanding spirituality. First, there is a professional discourse which is characterised by a belief that spiritual care is an important aspect of holistic care which is applicable to all patients, irrespective of their religious beliefs, which practitioners ought to provide. Most nurses would subscribe to this view. However, this is contrasted with a public discourse, expressed by most patients, who understood spirituality primarily to be a religious phenomenon and were surprised to find that it had anything to do with nursing.

It is important to note that the nurses and patients interviewed by McSherry understood the concept of spirituality in very different ways: the nurses tended to see it a secular professional term, whereas the patients associated the word spirituality with religion. It must necessarily be the case that our clients and patients will be culturally diverse and may have widely differing religious and secular beliefs. It is therefore not difficult to see the need for sensitivity when addressing spiritual care. The implication of this spiritual assessment will be discussed in the last section of the chapter.

Religion, spirituality and older people

Robinson et al. (2003) suggest that ageing is an ambiguous process associated with physical decline while also being a time of personal growth and development. This apparent contradiction requires explanation. Much of the decline of ageing is associated with loss, for example decline in physical strength, deterioration in sensory function and an increased susceptibility to disease which may lead to dependency for some people. Similarly, the older person may experience social losses as a consequence of bereavement or loss of occupational role at retirement.

There is a significant body of literature exploring the function of religion in later life, and the roles of religion for older people. Jewell (1999, 2004) and MacKinlay (2001, 2006) are significant authors in this field.

Jewell (2004), writing from a Christian perspective as a former Pastoral Director of the Methodist Homes for the Aged Care Group, outlines a model of spiritual needs which, for some, are addressed through religious observance. The six elements of the model are isolation, in that many older people may go for some days without physical or verbal contact with another human being; affirmation, through finding a purpose in life; celebration of significant life events life; confirmation or the need for one's value to be recognised by others; reconciliation to other people and to God by the healing of memories, repairing friendships or seeking forgiveness; and integration in the sense of the various strands of life into a transcendent, meaningful whole.

MacKinlay (2006) observes that an important consequence of the ageing of multicultural and multifaith western societies is the growing numbers of Muslims, Buddhists, Hindus, Jews, as well as Christians and those who do not practise any faith. She suggests that it is important for those who work with older people to be aware of the needs for use of ritual, symbols and religious practices of people from a wide range of backgrounds. This does not imply that nurses need to be intimately familiar with the liturgies and rituals of all faiths, as this would clearly be unrealistic, although it is helpful to have a basic understanding of key issues such as rituals at the time of death, and in this respect resources such as Neuberger (2004) are invaluable; but what is certainly desirable is to understand the concept that in all faiths, ultimate meanings are commonly expressed through ritual, patterns of behaviour, particular forms of dress, veneration of significant objects and so on.

It should not be thought that symbol and ritual are exotic expressions that can only be understood by religious believers, for they are also common in the everyday secular world. As an example of a secular ritual, consider the patterned behaviour that is involved in gaining access to another person's house. One steps up to the front door, knocks or rings the bell and then waits for the door to be opened. Then, after an invitation to enter (the host says 'come in' and steps to one side), one is free to step over the threshold, taking care to wipe one's shoes on the mat. This ritual is not just an empty convention: to most British people, it displays respect for the host and her territory. It may be a useful exercise to think of a number of secular rituals, which may range in significance from sharing a cup of tea together, to celebrating a major life transition and to reflect on the behaviours involved and the meanings they convey.

Finally, in this section, it is noted that there is significant evidence that religious involvement is associated with positive health outcomes for older people. Two representative papers can be cited to substantiate this. The first is provided by Fry (2000), who investigated the role of religiosity, spirituality and personal meaning in life in the well-being of older people within various residential and community settings. Fry found that personal meaning, involvement in formal religion and spiritual practices were clearly associated with well-being, particularly for those living in 'institutional' settings.

In a similar study among older adults in hospital, Koenig *et al.* (2004) found that religiousness and spirituality were consistently associated with greater social support, fewer depressive symptoms, better cognitive function and greater cooperativeness.

Skills focus: Assessing for culturally sensitive care

One of the persistent themes in the spirituality literature is the assessment of spiritual need (Rawlings-Anderson, 2004; McSherry 2006). MacKinlay (2006) offers a range of tools including a simple structured questionnaire and group topics for spiritual reminiscence which could be used for this purpose. However, in this chapter, we have suggested that culture is an important element in spirituality, and it is clear that people from different cultural backgrounds may vary significantly in their understanding of spirituality and in the ways in which they express values and meanings through words and actions, symbols and rituals. Those who are sensitive to cultural difference will wish to respect the cultural position of others during the assessment of spiritual need and the provision of spiritual care, and one way of doing this is for each of us to be familiar and comfortable with our own spirituality and its location in culture.

The philosopher, Hans Georg Gadamer, provides a conceptual tool which can help us to understand the problem and how to address it. Gadamer (1975) suggests that each of us understands the world from the perspective of a horizon. Literally, the horizon is everything that can be seen from a particular place, and significantly, the horizon changes for those who move. The concept of horizon can be taken as a metaphor for the culture we inhabit (professionally, personally or in some other way). A white, male British nurse living and working in the 21st century will have a horizon: he will see the world in a particular way. This horizon may be similar to the horizon of those of his colleagues who are women, but because of the difference in gender, it is likely that there will also be differences.

At the end of this chapter, we invite you to reflect on your own 'spiritual horizon'. As you look out at the world, what have you gained from your culture that enables you to see the world as you see it? You may find it helpful to represent your horizon by drawing a large circle on a piece of paper. Inside the circle, draw or describe the things that you can see clearly; but leave room outside the circle for things that are not part of your field of vision. Now compare notes with a colleague. How many points of similarity and of difference are there in our pictures? How far would you have to move to see the world from a different point of view? How long would the journey take, and what resources would you need in order to make it?

Conclusion

In this chapter, we have outlined three issues which have a bearing on the mental health of older people in its widest sense, but whose importance often seems to be neglected: spirituality, culture and religion. These three dimensions interact in complex ways. The growing literature on spirituality and health emphasises some of the ways in which older people may respond to the existential challenges of loss, bereavement and change, and suggests possible approaches to the assessment of spiritual need and ways of coping. Culture can be understood as a 'lens' or a set of assumptions, which may be expressed in symbolic ways including language, art and ritual, which offer a 'worldview' or perspective on the world. Importantly, we have noted that professional culture may differ from the lay perspective and suggested that nurses should seek to be as familiar as possible with the contours of their own 'horizon'. Finally, we have discussed the importance of religion as a resource for affirmation, celebration, confirmation, reconciliation and integration of the many strands of life into a meaningful whole, and we have noted research linking religious observance with well-being.

References

Baker, D. (1978) *Attitudes of nurses to care of the elderly.* Unpublished Ph.D. thesis, University of Manchester.

Carr A (1988) Transforming grace, Harper & Row, San Fransisco, p. 203.

Coleman, C.L. (2006) From the Guest Editor – Spirituality: An ongoing search for meaning: implications for mental and physical health. *Issues in Mental Health Nursing* **27**, 113–115.

Confoy, M. (2002) The contemporary search for meaning in suffering. In: *Spirituality and Palliative Care* (B. Rumbold, ed.). Melbourne, Oxford University Press, p. 23–37.

Cornah, D. (2006) *The Impact of Spirituality on Mental Health a Review of the Literature.* London, The Mental Health Foundation.

Culliford L. (2002) Spiritual care and psychiatric treatment: and introduction. *Advances in Psychiatric Treatment* **8**, 249–261.

Department of Health (2001a) *Your Guide to the NHS.* London, Department of Health.

Department of Health (2001b) *National Service Framework for Older People.* London, Department of Health.

Draper, P. (1994) *Promoting the quality of life of elderly people in nursing home care: a hermeneutical approach.* Unpublished Ph.D. thesis, University of Hull.

Dunn, D. (2004) Hearing the story: spiritual challenges for the ageing in an acute mental health unit. In: *Ageing, Spirituality and Well-Being* (A. Jewell, ed.). London, Jessica Kingsley.

Fry, P. (2000) Religious involvement, spirituality and personal meaning for life: existential predictors of psychological well-being in community-residing and institutional care elders. *Aging and Mental Health* **4** (4), 375–387.

Gadamer, H.G. (1975) *Truth and Method.* London, Sheed & Ward.

Golsworthy, R. and Coyle, A. (1999) Spiritual beliefs and the search for meaning among older adults following partner loss. *Mortality* **4** (1), 21–40.

Greasley, P., Chiu, L. F. and Gartland, M. (2001) The concept of spiritual care in mental health nursing. *Journal of Advanced Nursing* **33** (5), 629–637.

Haight, B. K., Christ, M. A. and Dias, J. K. (1994) Does nursing education promote ageism? *Journal of Advanced Nursing* **20**, 382–390.

Helman, C.G. (2001) *Culture, Health and Illness*, 4th edn. London, Arnold.

Jewell, A. (ed.) (1999) *Spirituality and Aging.* London, Jessica Kingsley.

Jewell, A. (ed.) (2004) *Ageing, Spirituality and Well-Being.* London, Jessica Kingsley.

Koenig, H., George, L. and Titus, P. (2004) Religion, spirituality and health in medically ill hospitalized older patients. *Journal of the American Geriatrics Society* **52**, 554–562.

MacKinlay, A. (2001) *The Spiritual Dimension of Ageing.* London, Jessica Kingsley.

MacKinlay, A. (2006) *Spiritual Growth and Care in the Fourth Age of Life.* London, Jessica Kingsley.

MacKinlay, A. and Cowan, S. (2003) Student nurses' attitudes towards working with older patients. *Journal of Advanced Nursing* **43** (3), 298–309.

MacKinlay, E.B. (1998) *The spiritual dimension of ageing: meaning in life, response to meaning and well-being in ageing.* Unpublished doctoral thesis, Melbourne, LaTrobe University.

McLafferty, I. and Morrison, F. (2004) Attitudes towards hospitalized older adults. *Journal of Advanced Nursing* **47** (4), 446–453.

McSherry, W. (2004) *The meaning of spirituality and spiritual care: an investigation of health care professionals, patients, and public's perceptions.* Unpublished Ph.D. thesis, Leeds Metropolitan University.

McSherry, W. (2006) *Making Sense of Spirituality in Nursing and Health Care Practice*, 2nd edn. London, Jessica Kingsley.

Melia, K. (1987) *Learning and Working: the Occupational Socialisation of Nurses.* London, Tavistock.

Narayanasamy, A. (2001) *Spiritual Care: A Practice Guide for Nurses and Health Care Practitioners*, 2nd edn. London, Quay Books.

Neuberger, J. (2004) *Caring for People of Different Faiths*, 3rd edn. Oxford, Radcliffe Medical Press.

Nolan, P. and Crawford, P. (1997) Towards a rhetoric of spirituality in mental health care. *Journal of Advanced Nursing* **26**, 289–294.

Rawlings-Anderson, K. (2004) Assessing the cultural and religious needs of older people. *Nursing Older People* **16** (8): 29–33.

Robinson, S., Kendrick, K. and Brown, A. (2003) *Spirituality and the Practice of Healthcare.* Houndsmill, UK, Palgrave Macmillan.

Swinton, J. (2001) *Spirituality and Mental Health Care Rediscovering a 'Forgotten' Dimension.* London, Jessica Kingsley.

Thomas, S.P. (2006) From The Editor – Introduction of the Special Issue, 'Spiritual And Religious Activities: Implications For Improving Mental Health', and the Guest Editor, Christopher Lance Coleman. *Issues in Mental Health Nursing* **27**, 111–112.

Webb, M. (2004) Spirituality in mental health. *Maryland Nurse* **6** (2), 7.

Chapter 10
Intimacy, Sex and Sexuality

Denise Forte, Diane Wells and Angela Cotter

Introduction

Older people's sexuality has received limited attention in the literature and even less in institutional care settings. Many in society see older people as asexual, and so sexuality is not an issue that receives much attention when assessing the health and social care needs of older people. This is especially true for gay, lesbian and bisexual older people and for those with a mental health condition, particularly dementia (Harris and Weir, 1998; Ward et al., 2005).

However, the reality challenges these ageist and negative stereotypes. Studies suggest that, although there may be a modest decline in sexual functioning with age, older people generally remain sexually active. In a study of 70-year-old women and men in Sweden, Persson (1980) found that men who continued to have sexual intercourse slept better and had better mental activity and a more positive attitude towards sexual activity in old age. Similarly, women who continued to have sexual intercourse retained their former levels of emotional stability, had lower levels of anxiety, had better mental health, felt generally more healthy and had a positive attitude towards sexual activity in old age (Persson, 1980; Ward et al., 2005).

Evidence suggests that sexual activity in younger age is a reasonable determinant of sexual activity in old age (Kessel, 2001). Additionally, in heterosexuals, any decline in sexual activity in a couple in old age is more frequently associated with the physical or mental health of the male rather than the female partner (Davies et al., 1998). Some studies support the view that age and sexual activity remain constant, but there is less information on the impact of mental health problems on sexual activity and satisfaction in older people (Davies et al., 1998) and even less if the older person is gay, lesbian or bisexual (Gott, 2005). Gott (2005) suggests that there is a tendency to regard all older people as heterosexual, despite the fact that 10% of the population is non-heterosexual, and older people are no different. The result is that the lived experience of older non-heterosexual people is missing from research, policy and practice (Gott, 2005), and their sexual needs go unmet, which is an even bigger problem for the older person and their partner if the person also has a mental health condition.

Given the general attitudes, it is not surprising that practitioners may feel at a loss in relation to supporting the sexuality of older people, especially those with a mental health need. As Clifford (2000) said, 'There is a proper shyness about sexuality' which influences practitioners, too and which spills over into their practice.

This chapter aims to:

- discuss the literature on sexuality, sexual problems and the importance of intimacy, sexuality and attachment in older people with mental health needs;
- discuss the skills required to enable people with mental health needs to experience intimacy and sexuality in a way that is appropriate for the older person and their partners and friends.
- discuss the support needed by health and social care staff so that they no longer feel at a loss when supporting older people with mental health needs to express their sexuality.

The backdrop to understanding relationships, intimacy and sexuality

Relationships that older people form whether intimate or sexual are often seen as divorced from the general context of relationships in life. Put simply, we all bring our past experience of relationships into each new relationship. So, as has been famously said, when two people meet, there are at least four others in the room – the parents of the two people as well. The importance of childhood relationships with parents in framing how we form later attachments has been recognised since the early days of psychoanalysis and is now common currency. Of particular relevance for older people's care is the knowledge that early child-hood experiences of loss of, or separation from, parents play an important role in how we meet later experiences of both loss and separation (Bowlby, 1973, 1980).

There are two ways that this theory can be useful to a consideration of older people's relationships and in particular those with a mental health needs. First, it is helpful because it gives a framework within which older people and staff can understand their own and each other's difficulties in making relation-ships and forming new attachments. Second, it is useful, too, because many older people may have been children who experienced separation from their parents through, for example, evacuation during the Second World War or through being hospitalised for an illness such as scarlet fever. It may help staff to understand some of the behaviour that older people show when they are sur-rounded by the experiences of loss than can accompany ageing, such as loss of a sexual partner or of intimate friends (Bowlby, 1988).

What do we mean by intimacy and sexuality?

Intimacy and sexuality are interrelated concepts, and any definition needs to reflect this. A number of definitions talk about the humanness of the individual including the need for closeness, identity and expressions of intimacy. Grigg (1999) suggests that it is through relationships that identity or sense of self is sustained. With all the changes that are liable to take place in later life, relationships are particularly important. They can provide comfort and support a sense of self/identity, especially during times of loss. This can be a loss of friends or family, or loss of function and independence. It is through our relationships that we understand and come to value friendships and love. Within this, however, long-term one-to-one sexual relationships, in whatever context, usually remain a valued part of the life experience. From this, it can be seen how important intimacy and sexuality remain for people with mental health needs where there is likely to be a loss of identity because of the illness itself.

When sexuality is understood as an integral aspect of each person's personality, it becomes easier to address this aspect of the person's life sensitively and in a way which allows for the many different forms of sexual expression that make up the rich fabric of society. Human sexuality is expressed in a variety of ways through personal-grooming habits, dress, touch, physical affection, companionship and the personalisation of one's environment as well as more sexually explicit behaviours.

As relationships form the fabric of identity, it is important to consider the different relationships making up the life of the older person and how these can be supported and encouraged when someone has a mental health condition such as depression, schizophrenia, bipolar disorder, alcohol or drug misuse or dementia. Relationship-centred care is an important part of any approach to supporting intimacy and sexuality in people with mental health needs. Sheard (2004) defines this as 'an inclusive approach that sees the person … within the context of important and significant relationships'.

When someone has a mental health need, this may affect the mutuality of the relationship. As one person in a couple relationship is cared for by the other, the relationship feels unequal in many respects. There can however be equality in moments of intimacy as each delights in a touch or a look which may contribute to a feeling of partnership (Hudson 2003).

Consider the example given in Case Study 10.1.

Case study 10.1

In a care home a couple of residents, Les and Mary, had formed a very intimate relationship despite both suffering from cognitive impairment as a result of alcohol misuse. In Les's case, this had been from a young age, but Mary's drinking had only begun in her fifties. Both have limited verbal skills. The researcher observing the interaction between Les and Mary was impressed with the level of non-verbal communication which demonstrated the reciprocity in the relationship, for example when one of them was telling a story or answering a question, they would seek verification from the other person, who in turn responded with smiles and nods.

It is important that staff and carers learn to recognise and value these moments of intimacy that enliven the days of older people including those with a mental health needs so that it also becomes a shared experience for both the person with the illness and those with whom they interact. It is worth highlighting the importance for this recognition to extend to all sexual relationships whether heterosexual or non-heterosexual.

A case study by Hellstrom et al. (2005) explored the way a relationship was maintained by a couple living with dementia. The story illustrated the role each of them had in maintaining the intimacy of their relationship. Much of the work of the carer was to maintain the identity of his wife by supporting her to continue to function in an effective way within the relationship. The study reported on the mutual love and support in the relationship and demonstrated a very skilled carer with the insight to empathise with his wife. The same skills and love are needed for partners when they are caring for someone they love with depression, schizophrenia, bipolar disorder, alcohol misuse or any other mental health condition, and it is up to health-care professionals to recognise and value the skills carers employ in supporting their loved ones in what can often be very stressful times. Older people with mental health needs in care homes may find themselves isolated from their loved ones because staff have failed to support the relationship the person came into the home with (Smyer and Qualls, 1999; Gott, 2005). Carers or partners may feel they need the permission of the staff to re-engage in the intimacy and activities they did at home.

Another study by Ward et al. (2005) took place in five care homes and involved recording the interactions that occurred in the public spaces between residents, staff and relatives. The research included the use of videos and care diaries. They observed that residents demonstrated warmth, closeness and intimacy among themselves, with same-sex friendships being the norm. Only one female and one male resident were seen to socialise regularly in an intimate way. The environment was found to play an important part in whether the residents engaged in intimacy or not. In some of the environments, there was a lack of space and opportunity for intimacy and sexual activity to take place, much of the activity occurring in public spaces. Seating generally in homes does not encourage closeness, as people sit around in high-backed chairs. However, intimacy and friendships appeared to be encouraged in the homes where individual chairs were supplemented with sofas. In another study, sitting on a sofa enabled two people with dementia to function as a couple validating each other through non-verbal communication.

As this study found, documentation for residents tends to refer to sexuality if it is deemed problematic. There was little evidence that any assessment of the sexual needs of the residents had been carried out, and any evidence of sexualised behaviour was reframed as part of the mental health illness. Sexual behaviour was often labelled as disinhibition and a problem. The documentation also highlighted concern for the vulnerability of female residents because of their cognitive impairment. Ward et al. (2005, p. 58) suggest that 'both types of concern highlight the role of care worker and wider organisation as regulator and monitor of residents' sexuality'. This position needs to be challenged if older people with mental health problems are to be enabled to lead a sexually active life as they desire.

Effects of age changes on sexuality

The research demonstrates that generally interest in sexuality remains high in older people and sexuality in old age can be seen as a developmental task of that part of the lifecycle (Benbow and Jagus, 2002, p. 263).

Ward et al. (2005) argue that we need to pay more attention to the part sexuality and sexual activity play in maintaining a gendered identity in ageing and how changes in rules governing sexuality throughout life impact on an individual's sexuality in older age.

However, a number of changes which may impact on the way the older person experiences sexual activity do occur with age. In women, there may be a lack of available partners, and they may have to rely on masturbation to relieve sexual tension, although this is less satisfactory than coitus (Benbow and Jagus, 2002). Changes to the vagina with a shortening of the vagina due to atrophy and a reduction in vaginal lubrication may mean that there is pain on intercourse or they are more prone to vaginal bleeding and infection. Sexual arousal is generally slower, and the intensity of the four phases is reduced, with fewer orgasmic contractions (Benbow and Jagus, 2002).

In men, with increasing age, there is a reduction of testosterone and erections which are not as full, orgasms tend to be briefer and the refractory period is longer, reducing the possibility of multiple erections (Jagus and Benbow 2002).

Intimacy and sexuality – issues for older people with mental health needs

Both organic and functional mental health disorders can cause problems with sexuality. In patients suffering from depression, the primary effect on sexual activity is a loss of sexual interest and desire. Depression can also affect the ability in men to have an erection and in women to gain sufficient vaginal lubrication to prevent pain and discomfit. However, it may provide a sense of comfort and positive emotional and physical response, which eases the depression (Davies et al., 1998; Jagus and Benbow, 2002).

Older women in particular have been found to be at greater risk of sexually transmitted disease because of a lack of knowledge about the importance of safe sex (Whipple and Scura, 1996). Those with a mental illness such as alcohol abuse, bipolar disorder and schizophrenia, which may lead to impaired decision-making and perhaps increased sexuality and disinhibition, are at even greater risk. Staff need to be alert when assessing these older people that they may have a sexually transmitted disease which may need treatment.

The onset of dementia does little to erase sexuality, but.it may alter the way love is given and perceived by both the person with dementia and their partner. For some caregivers, the act of sexual intimacy provides support and reassurance in the face of the partners devastating illness. For some older people with dementia, remaining sexually active may be one way of maintaining role identity. As one person with dementia commented, 'I can no longer provide an income, make decisions, or take care of things; this is the only thing I have that I can still give to my wife' (Davies et al., 1998, p. 195). As they found in their study, the more the couple can maintain a sexual intimacy, the more likely it is that the quality of the relationship will endure. The results from this study have similar implications for people struggling with identity issues due to other mental health conditions.

Sexual problems are relatively common in dementia, although the subject fails to be addressed in assessment unless the caregiver raises the issue first. Sexuality is more noted in men, and sexual behaviour is more explicitly linked as sexual in men rather than in women. In women, staff often fail to see the behaviour for what it is, i.e. sexual behaviour. In dementia units, staff are more likely to consider women with dementia as being vulnerable and in need of protection rather than someone who derives pleasure from sex. Sexual activity is often seen as a challenging behaviour rather than the need for comfort intimacy and reassurance (Archibald, 2002).

Problems associated with sexuality in people with a mental health illness

These problems include:

- Problems with sexual modesty where the person is unable to recognise the need for privacy.
- Specific sexual behaviours such as masturbation or inappropriate touch, or use of sexual language.
- Changes in sexual patterns in a marriage – either too many demands for sex as the person has forgotten they have already had sex or a loss of libido and interest in the person with dementia or the carer
- Illicit relationships or the forming of new relationships in care homes as people with dementia find each other. This presents ethical dilemmas for staff and relatives as they debate the capacity of the couple to consent to sexual activity. Teitelman and Copolillo (2002) suggest that for some people with dementia, impaired judgement and limited awareness may mean that they are vulnerable and unable to achieve a fully informed decision when it comes to sexual activity with a partner. Older people need to be protected if they are unable to make an informed decision, but equally staff and carers need to be careful about making proxy decisions for the person when they are able to consent.

- Disinhibition, which is primarily associated with frontal-lobe dementia such as Picks disease, which is about 7% of all dementias.
- Hypersexuality.
- Physical illness such as diabetes.
- Sexual dysfunction resulting from medication.

(Davies et al., 1998; Archibald, 2002; Jagus and Benbow, 2002; Ward et al., 2005)

Skills and strategies for supporting intimacy and sexuality in older people with mental health problems

The way a person relates to others and how they present themselves in dress and behaviour often indicate important aspects of how they feel about themselves as sexual beings. Hence, observation is extremely important. While behaviour and dress can clearly be observed visually, so can relationships. How it feels to be close to someone is important but may be a tricky area to get into, especially if practitioners disagree. The question for staff is: what are we going to do about the feelings?

The value of observation is that practitioners can then describe how the situation is. Consider the example given in Case Study 10.2.

Case study 10.2

Sam Brown has been coming to the day centre for 3 months, having been referred on discharge from hospital following treatment for severe depression. He often appears to be quite sad, although he enjoys being with one or two close friends. When at the day centre, he sits quietly most of the time. With a great deal of encouragement, he engages with others. Recently, he has made attempts to be friendly with Ada and Irene, who have responded with slight amusement. It is not clear why, but perhaps they are embarrassed. We are trying to support the friendship and encourage Sam to express his feelings more openly.

The above example illustrates both the complexity and importance of acknowledging our own feelings in these situations. Perhaps one of the biggest dangers, even when observing, is in categorising, labelling or even finding fault with what is observed. Here, the main purpose of the observation is to understand. There may not be any diagnoses to be made in this area, and if others are not being harmed, then relationships often need support rather than questioning.

The brief observation above shows how tentative this work often is and how it sometimes relies on the staff member being happy with 'not knowing'. 'Not knowing' and having the confidence to 'not know' while supporting a client is an important skill for practitioners when caring for sexuality (Clifford, 2000). The staff member did not know 'the answers', but they did know that there was warmth in Sam Brown's demeanor.

Many practitioners have trained themselves to 'not notice' their own feelings in order to be objective and non-judgmental. The non-judgmental feature is always important and embedded into codes of practice. Nevertheless, the objective feature can cause problems, as staff are expected and want to be empathic. This aspect of practice relies on having an emotional response. Empathy is 'having the capacity to put oneself in another's shoes'. Feelings are an important part of care delivery, but we need to use our own self-awareness to understand them.

Consider the example in Case Study 10.3.

Case study 10.3

John was an 86-year-old man suffering from moderate dementia when he moved into the local care home. He had only been there for 3 weeks when staff noticed he was becoming very friendly with Nora, a 70-year-old resident also with moderate dementia. One night, staff found John and Nora in bed together and were concerned as to how able Nora was to give informed consent to sexual intimacy.

The staff's initial reaction was to separate the couple, but they decided, as both were asleep and appeared comfortable, that they would leave it to the day staff to make a decision. They sought support from John and Nora's family as well as utilising the guidelines developed in the Providence Centre, a care home in Canada. These suggest that the first step in assessing questions of sexuality is for staff to examine their own attitudes towards sexuality and challenge any negative beliefs. The process is in three stages – a team meeting, a family meeting if necessary and ongoing assessment. The goal is to provide an objective assessment of the relationship.

They ask seven questions:

- What is the nature of the relationship?
- Are there any risks resulting from the behaviour and for whom?
- Is the behaviour causing distress or conflict of values for anyone, and if so why?
- What are the benefits of the relationship for both partners?
- Do the benefits outweigh the risks?
- Is there any evidence that either participant is not consenting to the relationship?
- Do those involved have the ability to understand the situation and to make decisions in light of that understanding (Doyle et al., 1999)?

If John and Nora can understand the situation and are both consenting, they have the right to privacy and liberty in forming their intimate relationship, including pursuing sexual activities of their choice, as long as the rights of other people are not compromised. Staff need to feel comfortable in supporting John and Nora's decision. If there is evidence that either John or Nora is not consenting to the relationship, they need to be supported in withdrawing from the relationship. Finding other ways to meet the needs for affection, self-esteem and intimacy through activities, touch or even a stuffed toy may be all that is needed. The tendency in such situations is to move one person to a new geographical location, but as Kuhn (2002) says, there has been little research on the effects of such moves on residents.

In an article by Teitelman and Copolillo (2002) about consent, they suggest the use of guidelines developed by Lichtenberg and Strzepek, which provides a way of determining if John and Nora are able to consent to having a sexual relationship. They look at three areas: awareness of the relationship, ability to avoid exploitation and awareness of potential risk. Under each of the three areas, they provide a subsidiary list of questions including, under risks, the risk of sexually transmitted disease. These guidelines are equally applicable for any older person with a mental health problem where there is some ambiguity as to whether the person is able to give informed consent.

Staff support and awareness

The above two examples demonstrate how tricky it is for staff to work effectively in supporting older people with mental health needs and their partners to maintain close personal relationships including sexual relationships which in turn foster dignity, identity and self-esteem in both partners of the relationship. Kitwood characterised the good member of staff as someone who has 'the ability to be emotionally "on the level" ... without the defensive "us and them" divisions that are so often found in the contexts of formal care' (Kitwood, 1995, p. 141).

Staff may unknowingly exacerbate the threats to residents' identity or sense of self, because of their own need to do things for people in order to feel whole themselves, and so a sense of self-awareness is critical. Fielo and Warren (1997) suggest for staff to be in a position to meet Kitwood's criteria and provide sensitive and empathetic care they need to:

- be aware of own attitudes regarding age and sexuality, and intervene with older people empathetically;
- know the changes with age in sexual response patterns and convey this information, as appropriate, to the older person;
- identify drugs that list sexual dysfunction as a side effect and design strategies to eliminate the adverse effects;
- understand the effects of illness on sexual expression and assist the older person in adapting to change;
- understand the effect of urinary incontinence on self-esteem and design strategies to promote continence;
- be aware that the lack of partners influences sexual fulfilment and help the older person increase social contact;

- work closely with significant others and health-care professionals in designing a plan that recognises the inter-relationship of all aspects of life, ensuring this remains part of any assessment;
- understand it is as important to support an older person's interest in sexual experience as it is to support their lack of interest in sexual experience (Fielo and Warren, 1997, p. 63).

They also suggest the need for more staff support in the form of group discussion and supervision. One such means is the Balint style seminar in which a consistent group of practitioners meet regularly to discuss examples of recent practice. One person opts to give a narrative account of a recent interaction with a client, from memory to the rest of the group. They listen carefully, trying to understand the practitioner/patient relationship, and very importantly the impact that the work has on the practitioner. First, it is training in self-awareness, and second it uses the psychodynamic principle that the feelings aroused in the practitioner might be related to the patient's world (Balint, 1964). Such awareness and scrutiny can take place in a supportive environment, and this approach can promote the therapeutic use of feelings and help with developing empathy.

Conclusion

This chapter has raised a number of key issues related to older people with mental health needs and their sexuality. It challenges the ageism that still persists in this area and draws on the literature to support the need for greater recognition of the importance of intimacy and sexuality in the lives of older people. A large emphasis has been on the importance of relationship-centred care in creating an environment where older people, their partners and friends feel safe in being open about their identity, sexual orientation and the relationships that are important to them, and where practitioners have developed the empathy to recognise and support them.

Resources

Age Concern England Campaign called Stonewall for Gay, Lesbian, Bisexual and Transgender Older People. Information can be found at the website: www.stonewall. org.uk/beyond_barriers/information/multiple_discrimination/800.asp
Alzheimer's Society Gay and Lesbian Carers Network: www.alzheimers.org.uk/carers/ gay Distance Learning Package
Archibald, C. and Chapman, A. (2005) *Sexuality and Dementia: a Guide for Staff Working with Dementia (Training Package)*. Dementia Services Development Centre, University of Stirling, e-mail dementia@stir.ac.uk or www.dementia.stir.ac.uk
Association of Psychosexual Nursing at www.associationpsychosexualnursing.org.
Balint Society www.balint.co.uk

References

Archibald, C. (2002) Sexuality and dementia in residential care – whose responsibility? *Sexual and Relationship Therapy* **17** (3), 301–309.

Balint, M. (1964) The Doctor, his Patient and the Illness. Edinburgh, Churchill Livingstone.

Benbow, S. and Jagus, C. (2002) Sexuality in older women with mental health problems. *Sexual and Relationship Therapy* **17** (3), 262–270.

Bowlby, J. (1973) *Separation: Anxiety and Anger*: Vol. 2 of Attachment and Loss. London, Hogarth Press.

Bowlby, J. (1980) *Loss: Sadness and Depression.* Vol. 3 of Attachment and Loss. London, Hogarth Press.

Bowlby, J. (1988) *A Secure Base: Clinical Applications of Attachment Theory.* London, Routledge.

Clifford, D. (2000) The courage to listen. In: *Caring for Sexuality in Health and Illness* (D. Wells, D. Clifford, M. Rutter, and J. Selby, J., eds). Edinburgh, Churchill Livingstone, pp. 335–362.

Davies, H., Zeiss, A., Shea, E. and Tinklenberg, J. (1998) Sexuality and intimacy in Alzheimer's patients and their partners. *Sexuality and Disability* **16** (3), 193–203.

Doyle, D., Bisson, D., Janes, N., Lynch, H. and Martin, C. (1999) Human sexuality in long term care. *Canadian Nurse* **95**, 26–29.

Fielo, S. and Warren, S. (1997) Sexual expression in a very old man: A nursing approach to care. *Geriatric Nursing* **18** (2), 61–64.

Gott, M. (2005) *Sexuality, Sexual Health and Ageing.* Milton Keynes, UK, Open University Press.

Grigg, E. (1999) Sexuality in older people. *Elderly Care* **11** (7), 12–15.

Harris, L. and Weir, M. (1998) Inappropriate sexual behavior in dementia: A review of the treatment literature. *Sexuality and Disability* **16** (3), 205–217.

Hellstrom, I., Nolan, M. and Lundh, U. (2005) We do things together. *Dementia* **4** (1), 7–22.

Hudson, R. (2003) *Dementia Nursing: A Guide to Practice.* Melbourne, Radcliffe Medical Press, pp. 225–234.

Jagus, C. and Benbow, S. (2002) Sexuality in older men with mental health problems. *Sexual and Relationship Therapy* **17** (3), 271–279.

Kessel, B. (2001) Sexuality in the older person. *Age and Ageing* **30**, 121–124.

Kitwood, T. (1995) Positive long term changes in dementia: some preliminary observations. *Journal of Mental Health* **4**, 133–144.

Kuhn, D. (2002) Intimacy, sexuality and residents with dementia. *Alzheimer's Care Quarterly* **3** (2), 165–176.

Persson, G. (1980) Sexuality in a 70 year old urban population. *Journal of Psychosomatic Research* **24**, 335–342.

Sheard, D. (2004) Person centred case: the emperor's new cloths? *Journal of Dementia Case* Mar/Apr 12(2), 22–24.

Smyer, M. and Qualls, S. (1999) *Ageing and Mental Health.* Oxford, Blackwell.

Teitelman, J. and Copolillo, A. (2002) Sexual abuse among persons with Alzheimer's disease. *Alzheimer's Care Quarterly* **3** (3), 252–257.

Ward, R., Vass, A., Aggarwal, N., Garfield, C. and Cybyk, B. (2005) A kiss is still a kiss? The construction of sexuality in dementia care. *Dementia* **4** (1), 49–72.

Whipple, B. and Scura, K. (1996) HIV in older adults. *American Journal of Nursing* **96**, 23–28.

Chapter 11
Nutrition

Christine Eberhardie

Introduction

Over the past 15 years, there has been a growing concern within health care that malnutrition, in the form of under- and overnutrition, is playing a very significant role in the cause of physical and mental ill health as well as being an impediment to successful treatment and outcome (Edington et al., 1996; Kelly et al., 2000). Undernutrition takes priority, but the effect of a diet high in saturated fats, salt and additives is resulting in an increase in hypertension and vascular dementia as well as diabetic-related depression.

Nutrition is an essential part of physical and mental health. Nutrition is required not only for physical energy, strength and stamina but also for mood, behaviour, motivation and relaxation. This chapter aims to:

- discuss the importance of nutrition in mood and behaviour;
- discuss the role of nutrition in the clinical management of dementia and depression;
- discuss the skills required to optimise the patient's nutrient intake.

Nutrients and the brain

The neurone is the functional unit of the brain. Each neurone communicates with other neurones by electrical and chemical neurotransmission in the potential space known as the synaptic cleft. Chemical neurotransmitters are released by the neurone into the synaptic cleft and selectively taken up by receptors on neighbouring neurones. This event is known as a synapse.

There are over 100 neurotransmitters, but some are so important that they have been the focus of neurochemical research for decades. One of the most well researched is the inhibitory neurotransmitter serotonin (5-hydroxytryptamine) and its role in mood, biological rhythms, food craving and seasonal affective disorder (Bonner and Waterhouse 1996).

Neurotransmitters require vitamins and essential amino acids from the protein in the diet for synthesis to take place. For example, serotonin cannot be synthesised without sufficient tryptophan in the diet. The best sources of tryptophan are turkey, chicken, tuna, soya, prawns and beef. There is some evidence to suggest that its uptake is enhanced by the presence of carbohydrate.

Research studies suggest that fish oils rich in omega-3 and omega-6 fatty acids, folate, folic acid, complex carbohydrates and vitamins B, C and E are required for a healthy brain (Van de Weyer, 2005). These nutrients are not a cure for organic brain disorders or mental illness, but there is a suggestion that they can help to prevent dementia and depression. They can also contribute to a successful outcome when a diet rich in these nutrients is given alongside conventional drug and psychotherapy.

What is a healthy diet, and where does it come from? In recent years, there has been a growing anxiety about the sources of food or 'the Food System' as Tansey and Worsley (1995) describe it. The Mental Health Foundation (2006) and Sustain (Van de Weyer, 2005), an alliance for better food and farming, have both produced reports campaigning for greater information about and monitoring of the system of food production and food standards. They also demonstrate the need for more research into the long-term accumulative effects of diet on the brain and mental health.

No one aspect of treatment and care can be seen in isolation. Drug therapy, environment, lifestyle, counselling and psychotherapy all play their part, and there is a need for more research that looks at the ways in which they combine to help or hinder care for mentally ill older people. A good example would be drug–nutrient and nutrient–nutrient interactions, especially in an age when more and more people are taking over-the-counter food supplements and herbal remedies.

Nutrition is not just a question of nutrients. It is also an inextricable part of personal, social, cultural and religious communication and ritual. Having a cup of coffee with a friend or a religious festival meal such as at Christmas, Ede or Diwali can be an important opportunity for the development and maintenance of relationships.

Assessment of nutrition and eating skills

There is a need for holistic and thorough assessment of nutritional factors which may affect the older person with mental illness of any kind. Much of what follows about dementia or depression can be used for other mental illnesses, in order to optimise the intake of an adequate and appropriate diet. The assessment should be multidisciplinary and interprofessional. The findings should also be available to all members of the care team. The assessment should include:

- nutritional status;
- food acquisition, storage and preparation skills;
- swallowing safety;
- eating skills;
- other functional ability;
- mental health status;
- environmental factors.

Nutritional status

There are several nutritional assessment tools available for use in the older adult, but the two which are well documented for their validity and reliability are the Mini Nutritional Assessment (Guigoz et al., 1994) and the Malnutrition Universal Screening Tool (MUST) developed by the British Association for Parenteral and Enteral Nutrition (2005). All of the assessments are based on the recording of height, weight and body mass index (BMI).

Calculating the BMI can be difficult in severely mentally ill patients, as the patient's cooperation is needed for accurate measurement. Normally, the patient would be measured standing upright under a stadiometer and weighed using a set of balance, bathroom or chair scales.

If the patient cannot stand upright, height can be calculated using armspan. The tape measure is placed from the sternal notch to the tip of the middle finger, and the resulting figure is doubled. Once the height is obtained, a patient can be weighed using a hoist, some of which are fitted with the means of calculating the BMI.

The Mini Nutritional Assessment tool is divided into two parts. The first part is a general screening for risk, and the second part is a more detailed assessment of a number of criteria, which would affect the patient's nutritional status including dentition, cognitive status and mobility. MUST is a tool for general use in adults and attempts to estimate the risk of malnutrition by a three-step approach:

- Step 1 calculates the body mass index, recording any unintentional weight loss in the last 3–6 months and any history of decreased food intake, loss of appetite or swallowing difficulties and psychosocial and physical disabilities which may contribute to weight loss.
- Step 2 is a series of calculations involving all the parameters outlined in Step 1 to give an overall risk score.
- Step 3 is the management of the risk and a plan of care (British Association for Parenteral and Enteral Nutrition 2000).

Nurses can play a key role in screening and referral to the dietician. It is also important to take note of any food allergies and intolerances as well as any food supplements, over-the-counter remedies and complementary treatments the patient takes. It is not unusual today for people in their eighties to be taking aspirin, ginkgo biloba, vitamin E, magnesium and other supplements in an attempt to delay memory loss. More research is required into the accumulative effect of high doses of these nutrients on the brain.

Food acquisition, storage and preparation skills

The ability to search for food, choose it, prepare it for cooking and eating and to store dry or frozen food safely is a complex of sensory and psychomotor skills (Eberhardie, 2002). Some of these skills require an overview from a nurse, but a more specialised assessment by an occupational therapist and/or physiotherapist will be needed. The physiotherapist may assess the ability to get on and off buses, carry loads, reach food on upper or lower shelves, grasp an object and hold, open, or use equipment or containers safely.

Assessments made by occupational therapists usually involve assessing the ability to carry out tasks on home visits or in a kitchen within the rehabilitation unit. In care home settings, Wenborn (2003) suggests that cookery sessions can not only be a time for assessment but also stimulate memory and social interaction.

Swallowing safety

There are many reasons for swallowing problems in the older person from gastro-oesophageal reflux to stroke. Recent research studies show that nurses trained in clinical bedside assessment of swallowing can play a valuable part in preventing the complications of dysphagia and optimising nutritional support (Scottish Intercollegiate Guidelines Network, 2004). Signs of swallowing problems are poor lip closure, drooling, stiff tongue, gurgling speech and choking or coughing. The test involves giving a teaspoonful of water provided that the patient does not have any of the above signs. If there are no signs of distress the patient is given a teaspoon of water on two further occasions (Perry and Love, 2001). If the patient experiences any sign of distress, they should be referred to a speech and language therapist.

Eating-skills assessment

Before someone eats, they have to decide what they want to eat as well as when, how and where they want to eat it. The choice of food, the rituals of mealtimes and ways of eating, although individual, are influenced by culture and religion as well as social group. It is important to be aware of any food taboos the patient may have or views on food combining. Patients may also have particular health beliefs about certain foods.

Eating skills will also involve assessing the patient for the following potential problems:

- Limited arm movement which may affect the ability to lift cutlery to the mouth.
- Sensory processing difficulties which could lead to:
  - Visual or tactile agnosia (the inability to recognise objects by sight or touch).
  - Acquired dyspraxia (difficulty with perception and patterns of movement e.g. difficulty picking up a fork, putting food on it, and lifting it to the mouth).
  - One-sided neglect (the patient ignores one side of the body).
- Poor hand–eye coordination, ataxia (lack of coordination) or bradykinesia (slowness of movement) such as can be found in patients with Parkinson's disease.
- The speed at which the individual eats and the quantity of food they eat must also be monitored. Some patients with dementia may eat very quickly. Patients with depression often eat very slowly and very small amounts.

Other functional ability

There are many physical problems of old age that can affect the individual's desire to eat and drink such as diminished acuity of taste and smell, gastro-oesophageal reflux and feeling bloated. Continence also affects the patient's attitudes to choice of food and fluids. Fear of incontinence of urine or faeces can lead to a patient's refusing food and fluids. A tendency to constipation and diarrhoea can also affect the desire to eat and choice of food.

Mental health status

The patient's mental state can be assessed using appropriate assessment tools which can be used by clinical psychologists or, in some cases, other members of the multidisciplinary team. Tools such as the Mini Mental State Examination (2001) are useful to assess cognitive changes or the Geriatric Depression Scale (Sheikh and Yesavage, 1986) to assess depression. Other aspects of eating behaviour which need to be recorded are pica (inappropriate or dangerous objects, e.g. coal or hair gel), frenzied eating or food refusal.

Backstrom *et al.* (1987) showed that nutritional intake improved if the numbers of people who fed the patient were reduced, enabling a rapport to build up between the nurse or nursing assistant and the patient.

Environmental issues

The environment in which the patient lives and takes meals needs to be uncluttered and the dining area easy to prepare. The changes which need to be made, to ensure that dementia patients are kept calm and encouraged to eat, will be addressed later in this chapter.

Nutritional issues in the clinical management of dementia

The type of dementia the patient has and how far it has progressed determine what form the clinical management takes. In the early stages, reminders to eat and drink may be sufficient, and some patients may continue to have a good quality of life before their condition deteriorates.

Loss of memory brings with it dangers. Patients may forget to eat and drink, leave the gas on or let pans boil dry. Too much food may be bought and left to rot in the refrigerator. However, some simple measures can help to keep patients safe and independent for as long as possible. Clear the kitchen clutter, and try to maintain a regular routine for shopping, storing and cooking food.

As the disease progresses, the person will need more supervision, and meals need to be provided. In care homes and hospitals, it is important to continue a routine, and research shows that there should be a designated dining area with plain table cloths, the minimum of crockery and cutlery and no distractions like televisions or CD players. Some suggest that the tables should be round and seat no more than six people.

For those who have a very poor attention span and are very restless, hot meals may remain uneaten. For these patients, finger foods and energy-dense fortified snacks may be a better option, e.g. chicken drumsticks, sandwiches and crudités, or an omelette fortified with milk and cheese.

Those who are fast eaters need to be reminded to slow down, and those who eat very slowly need careful monitoring and an energy-dense diet (Kindell, 2002). In the advanced stages of the treatment, pica may occur. It is important to prevent the patients from harming themselves.

Eventually, the patient will require assistance with feeding, and nurses may wish to use the EDFEd2 scale developed by Watson (1994). This scale enables the nurse to identify and monitor the eating behaviour of the patient, e.g. food refusal, spitting and hoarding food in the mouth.

Good non-verbal communication calms anxious patients and builds trust (Le May, 2004), which encourages eating, since part of the food refusal is due to a clouding of consciousness and fear of being poisoned. A calm, gentle and smiling approach is reassuring and lessens the patient's anxiety.

There are ethical and legal issues which, in an ideal situation, should be addressed before the patient lacks the ability to make informed choices. One of these decisions is whether or not artificial feeding should be instituted when the patient is no longer able to take an oral diet.

This is a very difficult and sensitive area. Up to the time of writing, the withdrawal or withholding of treatment has been a doctor's decision following consultation with the family. From October 2007, the Mental Capacity Act will come into force. For more information and discussion of the Act, turn to Chapter 6.

Nutritional issues in the clinical management of depression

The reasons for depression are discussed in Chapter 16 but whether the depression is reactive or endogenous the sufferer's appetite may be affected. It is usually diminished and the patient eats little food. In some cases, the patient has little or no appetite for food; in others, they overeat. For some, the treatment affects appetite, and there is either weight gain or weight loss, e.g. lithium.

Some people fear the stigma of depression and seek over-the-counter preparations such as St John's Wort which, on its own, is relatively harmless but, when taken with selected serotonin-reuptake inhibitors (SSRI), can be lethal.

Reflection

The two clinical case studies (Alzheimer's type dementia in Case Study 11.1 and depresion in Case Study 11.2) offered aim to enable readers put the issues raised in this chapter into context.

Case study 11.1

James is 83 years old and has lived alone since his wife died 3 years ago. He has been admitted for assessment because he was found wandering in the street in the middle of the night. On admission, James has clearly been neglecting himself. He is very restless and agitated, and behaves in a very defensive manner, which is often aggressive. You are asked to measure James's weight and height, and calculate his BMI. What will you do if James refuses to be weighed and resists attempts to be measured? How will you encourage James to eat?

Case study 11.2

Jane, 77 years old, has been widowed for 3 months. Her daughter helped her for 6 weeks after the funeral but has gone back to her own family, as she thinks her mother is taking her for granted and becoming too dependent .

Jane stays at home. She takes a long time to get to sleep and wakes up early. Jane does not feel like eating, and the neighbour persuades her to call the GP and ask him to visit. Jane is found to have depression and is admitted to a psychiatric unit for assessment and treatment .

On admission, Jane is found to have a BMI of 18, sores on her lips, dry skin and pressure ulcers on her sacrum and hips. She remains very withdrawn.

How will you encourage her to eat? How will you restore her nutritional status?

Conclusion

Nutrition is very important in the maintenance of mental health and the prevention of some forms of dementia. It also plays a key role in the social, cultural and religious life of the individual. Holistic assessment of the patient involves more than just nutritional status. Appropriate assessment tools need to be used for this purpose, leading to interprofessional referrals. Good verbal and non-verbal communication skills can encourage patients to eat when they do not feel like it. The environment needs to be arranged in such a way as to minimise distractions and encourage eating.

References

Backstrom, A., Norberg, A. and Norberg, B. (1987) Feeding difficulties in long stay patients at nursing homes. Care giver turnover and caregivers' assessments of duration and difficulty of assisted feeding and amount of food received by the patient. *International Journal of Nursing Studies* **24**, 69–76.

Bonner, A.B. and Waterhouse, J. (1996) *Molecules to Mankind*. London, Macmillan.

British Association for Parenteral and Enteral Nutrition (2000) *Malnutrition Universal Screening Tool*. http://www.bapen.org.uk/pdfs/Must/must_full

Eberhardie, C. (2002) Nutrition and the older adult. *Nursing Older People* **14** (2), 20–25.

Edington, J., Kon, P. and Martyn, C.N. (1996) Prevalence of malnutrition in patients in general practice *Clinical Nutrition* **15**, 60–63.

Guigoz, Y., Vellas, B. and Garry, P.J. (1994) Mini-nutritional assessment: a practical assessment tool for grading the nutritional state of elderly patients. *Facts and Research in Gerontology* **4** (2), 5–59.

Kelly, I.E., Tessier, S., Cahill, A., Morris, S.E., Crumley, A., McLaughlin, D., McKee, R.F. and Lean, M.E.J. (2000) Still hungry in hospital: identifying malnutrition in acute hospital admissions. *Quarterly Journal of Medicine* **93**, 93–98.

Kindell, J. (2002) *Feeding and Swallowing Disorders in Dementia.* Bicester, UK: Speechmark.

Le May, A. (2004) Building rapport through non-verbal communication. *Nursing and Residential Care* **6** (10), 488–491.

Mental Health Foundation (2006) *Feeding minds: the impact of food on mental health.* http://www.mentalhealth.org.uk/html/content/feedingminds_report.pdf

Mini Mental State Examination (2001) http://www.nemc.org/psych/mmse.asp

Perry, L. Love, C. (2001) Screening and Assessment of dysphagia in acute stroke: a systematic review *Dysphagia* **16** (1), 1–12.

Scottish Intercollegiate Guidelines Network (2004) *Management of patients with stroke: Identification and management of dysphagia. No. 78.* http://www.sign.ac.uk/pdf/sign78.pdf

Sheikh, R.L. and Yesavage, J.A. (1986) Geriatric Depression Scale (GDS): recent evidence and development of a shorter version. *Clinical Gerontologist* **5**, 165–173.

Tansey, G. and Worsley, T. (1995) *The Food System. A Guide.* London, Earthscan.

Van de Weyer, C. (2005) *Changing Diets, Changing Minds: How Food Affects Mental Well-Being and Behaviour.* London, Sustain.

Watson, R. (1994) Measuring feeding difficulty in patients with dementia: replication and validation of the Edfed Scale #1. *Journal of Advanced Nursing* **19** (5), 850–855.

Wenborn, J. (2003) Incorporating food and drink into stimulating activities. *Nursing and Residential Care* **5** (7), 338–339.

Chapter 12
Palliative and End-of-Life Care

Lynne Phair

Introduction

Care at the end of a person's life as a specialist subject has, traditionally, focused on palliative care of people with cancer. The hospice movement was set up specifically for this purpose and campaigned to ensure that people dying of cancer received the specialist care they needed. Strategies for cancer services have been introduced over the last decade, but the Cancer Plan (Department of Health 2000) sets out the steps for improving services for prevention, early detection, quality treatment and supportive care for all (Morrison and Garland 2004), and demonstrates a commitment to providing palliative care for all patients with life-limiting illness (Evans and Walsh 2002).

The hospice movement and the Cancer Plan support only a small proportion of people who need end-of-life care. Causes of death are changing, more people die of circulatory disease (37%), respiratory disease (13%) and other non-specific conditions (19%), while cancer causes 27% of deaths (Eolc, 2006). Indeed, at the beginning of the 20th century, children aged 0–4 years were the age group with the highest proportion of deaths, but by 2004, 65% of all people who died were aged 75 or over (Age Concern, 2005).

In 2003, the Department of Health (England) launched the NHS End-of-life Care Programme. This is part of an overall strategy to address some of the challenges of enabling people to receive the care they want, and need, in the place of their choice. In 2002, the World Health Organisation defined palliative care as:

'an approach that improves the quality of life of patients and their families facing problems associated with life-threatening illness, through the prevention and relief of suffering by means of early identification and impeccable assessment and treatment of pain and other problems, physical, psychological and spiritual.' (World Health Organisation 2002)

Within the End-of-Life Care Programme, 'End-of-life Care' usually refers to the last 6–9 months of a person's life, and 'Terminal Care' is associated with the last few days or hours of life, once it is known that the person is dying.

Death and dying in today's society

Traditionally, in the UK, beliefs and attitudes towards death and dying have been very personal; it is not a subject the British traditionally discuss, and often plans have not been made in respect of the care and treatment a person wants at the end of their life. Funeral Plans are becoming more widely advertised, and the legislation in respect of advanced directives is changing. The concept of a 'good death' has been developed (Age Concern, 1999), and the House of Commons Health Committee inquiry into palliative care concluded that the right to a good death should be fundamental (House of Commons Health Committee 2004 in Age Concern, 2005). What is considered to be a good death will depend on a number of factors, including, culture, religion and spiritual belief, impact of the illness and the person's understanding, family and personal circumstances and opportunities available for support. In 1999, Age Concern identified the principles of a 'good death' as:

- to know when death is coming and to understand what can be expected;
- to be able to retain control of what happens;
- to be afforded dignity and privacy;
- to have control over pain relief and other symptoms management;
- to have choice and control over where death occurs (at home or elsewhere);
- to have access to information and expertise of whatever kind is necessary;
- to have access to any spiritual or emotional support as required;
- to have access to hospice care in any location, not only in hospital;
- to have control over who is present and who shares the end;
- to be able to issue advance directives, which ensure that wishes are respected;
- to have time to say goodbye and to have control over other aspects of timing;
- to be able to leave when it is time to go, and not have life prolonged pointlessly.

(Age Concern 1999 in Evans and Walsh, 2002).

The End-of-Life Care Programme has an aim to widen the pool of staff trained to support this client group. The documents Improving Supportive and Palliative Care for Adults with Cancer (National Institute for Health and Clinical Excellence (National Institute for Clinical Excellence 2003) have highlighted three examples of good practice:

- Gold Standards Framework;
- Liverpool Care Pathway;
- Preferred Place of Care.

We will apply these examples later in the chapter.

The challenges for mental health nurses working with people at the end of their lives

Working with older people who have mental health problems has not always ensured that mental health nurses have the physical skills required when a person is at the end of their life. Caring for a person at end-stage dementia is often translated as being 'basic' or 'social care', a view which can be reinforced by continuing health-care assessments or the overall lower funding given to the care of older people with palliative care needs as opposed to children or young adults who have palliative-care requirements. Other groups of mental health clients with enduring mental health problems, depression or even forensic mental health needs can be bypassed even more readily unless the predominant health condition becomes a physical need. Within General Forensic Secure environments, the number of older people is increasing, and inmates die, having required palliative care services, but often not receiving them (Fowler-Kerry, 2003). For people with enduring mental health problems, the long-term effects of high doses of psychotropic medication, the erosion of a person's social skills and ability to follow a positive approach to healthy life (e.g. not smoking or managing obesity), together with other complications including the possible high use of alcohol or substance misuse, all show that older people with all types of mental health conditions may need end-of-life care, which may need to be led by the mental health nurse.

Cutcliffe et al. (2001a, b) argue that mental health nurses focus and connect with people in their distress, providing security and human relationship where the person can search for meaning and truth. There are areas of commonality between palliative care nurses and mental health nurses, as both groups possess skills in psychological, social, spiritual and focus of control of the person, although they also identify a different approach in some aspects of practice, including facilitative or confrontational counselling and aspects of physical care. Mental health nurses do not generally have the physical/technical skills to undertake all aspects of the palliative care of their patients, but with the application of an open mind, there are a number of similarities and assessment skills which could mean that the two services could work more closely together.

The physical health of people with severe mental illness (SMI) is a continuing concern, and evidence shows that psychiatric patients have high rates of physical illness that go largely undetected. Nash (2005) believes that physical health problems, which can cause death, are exacerbated due to the sedentary lifestyles of people with SMI. There is also concern that sometimes symptoms are mistaken for aspects of mental illness, including symptoms common at the end of life, including increased pain, anoxia, weight loss and constipation. There is a difference of view within mental health nursing regarding the importance of knowledge of physical and medical health problems, and clinical skills tend to focus on those required for psychiatric interventions. Nash concludes that the philosophy of holistic care in mental health must embrace physical care needs, just as it embraces social, environmental, economic and psychological needs.

Assessing the needs of older people with mental health needs at the end of their lives

Most nurses who work in services for older people will believe that all assessments they carry out are person-centred. Thus, this principle should be applied to assessing the needs of End-of-life care. As stated in the National Service Framework for Older People (Department of Health, 2001), by taking a person-centred approach older people are treated as individuals, and they receive timely packages of care which meet their needs as individuals. The Registered Nurses assessment should ensure that this is achieved either by delivering the care personally or care-managing a package, and being involved as the nurse's expertise allows. Webster (2004) identifies that there are a number of factors that impede assessment and create an unsatisfactory outcome; these include:

- adhering to rigid and unbending frameworks or tools for assessment;
- task-focused or ritualistic practice;
- non-person-centred cultures and autocratic leadership;
- lack of creativity in practice.

Yet, Ford and McCormack (2000) argue that a key theme which emerges about the process of assessment with older people is a highly skilled, unique activity that requires expert knowledge of:

- the practice of caring for and working with individuals;
- an understanding of the social political context of ageing;
- an understanding of biological and psychological developments through the lifespan;
- an understanding of the needs of populations.

Meeting the challenges and offering appropriate care at the end of a person's life

The focus of the End-of-life Care programme is to develop the capabilities of generalist nurses. Thus, applying the principles of End-of-life Care to Older People with mental health problems who require palliative care will enhance and improve their quality of life and quality of care. Three examples from the National Institute for Clinical Excellence (2003) have been heralded as good practice to be used in any setting by non-specialist nurses.

The Gold Standards Framework (GSF)

This framework can be used when people are likely to be in the last 6–9 months of life. It has been designed for use in primary care and care homes and helps to manage symptoms by giving the older person and their family both involvement and confidence in their care.

The Liverpool Care Pathway for the dying Patient (LCP)

This tool has been developed in order to care for someone in the last days or hours of life, once it is known that the person is dying.

Preferred Place of Care (PPC) (Advanced Care Planning)

This project is an example of an advanced care plan and is a document which states the patient's preferred place of care, and type and intervention of care they prefer to receive.

Using the Gold Standard Framework

This programme has been designed to be led by a GP, but the principles can be applied by any health or social-care professional. The process of Goals and Key Tasks are not unfamiliar to any mental health worker who uses person-centred care as their philosophy of practice. The aim of the Gold Standard is to aspire that all patients nearing the end of life, whatever the diagnosis, stage or setting, receive the best of all care (Gold Standards Framework, 2005).

The process

- identify the patient's needs;
- assess their needs, symptoms, preferences and important issues;
- plan the care around the patient's needs and enable these to be fulfilled, in particular, where they want to live and die.

The goals

The person should:

- be symptom-free;
- be cared for, where they choose;
- have security and support – more information – less fear;
- have supported, informed and empowered family and carers;
- be cared for by confident, team-focused staff.

The key tasks – the 7C's

- C1 – communication;
- C2 – coordination;
- C3 – control of symptoms;
- C4 – continuity, including out of hours;
- C5 – continued learning;
- C6 – carer support;
- C7 – care in the dying phase.

Many of the principles of the Gold Standard apply to good care practice with people with every condition. The mental health nurse must think about how to apply their skills and knowledge, and work with others to promote positive palliative care. The mental health nurse may feel that they cannot contribute and so disengage, but this will not enable a Gold Standard of care. Collaborative working is vital, and ensuring all practitioners work with others is in the best interest of the older person. An example of palliative care in the community is given in Case Study 12.1.

Case study 12.1

John is 86 years old. He suffers from bipolar disorder, chronic obstructive airways disease, heart failure, and benign prostatic hyperplasia. He was becoming increasingly frail, confused, and reluctant to drink. His wife, as the main carer, was struggling to manage him. John was also supported by a community matron. On one visit, he was noted to be increasingly confused, verbally aggressive, not eating or drinking and breathless; he also had swollen ankles. The community matron diagnosed dehydration and a urinary-tract infection. She contacted the CPN requesting a joint visit and assessment, in order to use joint expertise to support John and his wife, to stabilise his condition and so to avoid a hospital admission. This scenario has two endings:

A Gold Standard response
The joint visit was undertaken and the CPN reviewed the medication in relation to his other conditions and used active listen and psychosocial communication skills to re-establish a therapeutic relationship. He identified non-confrontational techniques to ensure that antibiotics and fluids were taken, and agreed with John and his wife and the community matron, about the priorities of treatment and methods of enabling fluid intake. The community matron assessed the physical-health needs, and both professionals agreed a joint plan about how John could stay at home.

A traditional response
The CPN refused to go to see John, as his deteriorating mental health was due to his urinary-tract infection and so was not a mental-health problem. The community matron was unable to review and work with psychological approaches needed at the level required by John, and he had to be admitted to hospital.

The Liverpool Care of the Dying Pathway

This pathway has been developed to be used when a person is in the last days or hours of life (Marie Curie Cancer Care, 2006). The pathway is detailed and enables review every 2 hours. Indeed, goals for care can only be set for 2 hours, to ensure the care is focused and intensive. The patient focus of care includes pain, agitation, respiratory track secretions, dyspnoea, mouth care, nausea and vomiting and micturition difficulties. The care needs will depend on the condition the person is suffering from and the interrelationship between the physical and mental health condition. For many people, the GP will be able to administer appropriate medication, and mental health nurses who work with frail older people will have the skills in general physical care. This should be the case, as many complications of advanced and end-stage dementia are the conditions listed on the Liverpool Pathway. An example of the Liverpool Care Pathway is given in Case Study 12.2.

Case Study 12.2

Emily has lived at the Meadows Nursing Home for people with dementia for 3 years. She had deteriorated from being able to walk about and talk to, over the past 2 months, being unable to sit up unaided or respond to her name. The RMN had followed the Gold Standard Framework, and her physical, spiritual and psychological needs had been managed well with the support of the GP and the involvement of her family. Emily had curled up into the foetal position and grimaced when moved. Her pain was assessed using the DOLOPLUS 2 Scale (Wary et al., 1993), and a syringe driver was set up by the district nurse. Her favourite music was played quietly and her family encouraged to be with her. Her continence was managed with pads, she was turned 2–4-hourly and pressure risk was managed on a dynamic overlay, as identified in her assessment. She enjoyed small amounts of ice cream, and she had 4-hourly mouth care. Her family undertook hand massage and read passages of the bible to her (as she had a deep faith). As her symptoms changed, the nurses told the family what was happening and monitored for any signs of distress, sips of fluid were offered, but the nurse described how the lack of interest in fluids was part of the dying process at this stage. Emily died in the company of her daughter and pain-free.

Case Study 12.3

Phyllis has suffered with anxiety and depression for over 30 years. She has been under the care of a CPN and a psychiatrist for episodes during this time. She is a widow, and both her children live abroad. She has suffered from Parkinson's disease for about 10 years, which is now in the end stages. The CPN arranges a joint visit with the GP to discuss the impact of these two conditions and Phyllis's future needs and plans. The discussion, which is highly sensitive and requires a high level of communication skills, is tailored to her needs, including discussions about her preferences for a place of care, resuscitation or allowing a natural death agreement and also Lasting Power of Attorney information (Gold Standards Framework, 2005).

Advanced care planning

The third programme of good practice is in relation to the use of an Advanced Care Plan (ACP) with the older person and their carer. This is different from an Advanced Directive and enables discussion of more specific planning around the person's current needs.

Conclusion

Caring for older people and their families at the end of their life is just as important as at any other time. The mental health nurse has a responsibility to ensure that symptoms of an end-of-life condition are not misdiagnosed as a symptom of their mental health condition, and equally, the impact of any mental conditions on other physical illnesses should be assessed and reviewed co-terminously. Mental Health workers who work with older people must ensure that their knowledge and skills encompass more than those dictated by traditional nursing boundaries, and they must ensure that they work with other physical-health professionals so that older people with mental health needs truly receive Gold Standard care at the end of their lives.

References

Age Concern (1999) The Future Health and Care of Older People: The Best is Yet to Come. London, Age Concern.

Age Concern (2005) *Dying and Death. Policy Position Papers*. London, Age Concern.

Cutcliffe, J., Black, C., Hanson, E. and Goward, P. (2001a) The commonality and sychronicity of mental health nurses and palliative care nurses: Closer than you think? Part 1. *Journal of Psychiatric and Mental Health Nursing* **8**, 53–59.

Cutcliffe, J., Black, C., Hanson, E. and Goward, P. (2001b) The commonality and sychronicity of mental health nurses and palliative care nurses: Closer than you think? Part 2. *Journal of Psychiatric and Mental Health Nursing* **8**, 61–66.

Department of Health (2000) *The NHS Cancer Plan*. London, Department of Health. http://www.DH.gov.uk/cancerplan.htm

Department of Health (2001) *The National Service Framework for Older People*. London, Department of Health.

Eolc (2006) *NHS End-of-life Care Programme Progress Report*. March 2006. http://www.end-oflifecare.nhs.uk

Evans, N. and Walsh, H. (2002) The organisation of death and dying in today's society. *Nursing Standard* **16** (25), 33–38.

Ford, P. and McCormack, B. (2000) Keeping the person in the centre of nursing. *Nursing Standard* **14** (46), 50–44.

Fowler-Kerry, S. (2003) Palliative care within secure forensic environments. *Journal of Psychiatric and Mental Health Nursing* **10**, 367–369.

Gold Standards Framework (2005) *The Gold Standard Framework*. London, Royal College of General Practitioners. http://www.goldstandardsframework.nhs.uk

Marie Curie Cancer Care (2006) *Liverpool care pathway care of the dying pathway*. http://www.lcp.mariecurie.org.uk

Morrison, J. and Garland, E. (2004) Developing palliative care services in partnership. *Cancer Nursing Practice* **3** (3), 22–25.

Nash, M. (2005) Physical care skills: a training needs analysis of inpatient and community mental health nurses. *Mental Health Practice* **9** (4), 20–23.

National Institute for Clinical Excellence (2004) *Improving Supportive and Palliative Care for Adults with Cancer.*, London, National Institute for Clinical Excellence.

Wary, B. (1993) et ai. In Roy D, Rapin, C. (eds) Douleur etantalgie Les annales de soins palliatifs 89–98 in Murdoch, J. Larsen, D. (2004). Assessing pain in cognitively impaired older adults. *Nursing Standard* **18** (38), 33–39.

Webster, J. (2004) Person-centred assessment with older people. *Nursing Older People* **16** (3), 22–26.

World Health Organisation (2002) *National Cancer Control Programmes. Polices And Managerial Guidelines*, 2nd edn. Geneva, World Health Organisation.

Part 4
MENTAL HEALTH ISSUES FOR OLDER PEOPLE

Chapter 13
Acute Mental Health Issues

Sarah McGeorge

Introduction

This chapter explores behaviour which may be considered 'challenging' or 'disruptive', though this concept needs careful consideration, as it is important to ask for whom the behaviour is challenging. Kitwood (1997) suggested that in dementia care, all behaviour is an attempt to communicate. In order to explore these ideas, this chapter will examine theoretical models which seek to help us understand behaviour; factors which have been shown to cause or exacerbate such behaviour; approaches and interventions which may prevent or reduce, so-called problematic behaviour, and the skills which are necessary to provide nursing care to older people who are acutely distressed. The majority of research and academic writing about problematic behaviour in older people focuses on people with dementia, and emanates from the USA. There is little evidence to date relating to problematic behaviour in older people with mental health conditions other than dementia and this is an area that needs further attention and research. An example of a model, the Need-Driven Dementia Compromised Behaviour model (NDB) is illustrated with a short case study to demonstrate how a framework may assist you when working with older people who may provide a challenge through their behaviour.

The favoured term for such acute mental health issues in the UK is at present 'challenging behaviour', but it is evident from the literature that there are many other terms used synonymously: 'disruptive behaviour' (Bair et al., 1999; Gerdner et al., 2002); 'non-normative behaviour' (Kovach et al., 2005); 'behavioural expressions' (Chiu, 1991); 'behavioural disturbance' (Buhr and White, 2006); and most recently 'behaviour which challenges' (National Institute of Clinical Excellence, 2006). There is an inherent problem with these terms. Put simply, it is now recognised that terms such as 'challenging behaviour' carry with them negative connotations, which may lead to low expectations of individuals' abilities, and that these can influence the attitudes of carers (Chiu, 1991). Dewing (2005) also notes that descriptions of problematic behaviour can result in negative labelling of older people (e.g. 'the wanderer'). Other pejorative terms such as 'attention-seeking behaviour' and 'manipulative behaviour' are equally unhelpful but unfortunately sometimes still in use. The risk for nurses and older people is that, in using such terms, we will fail to see beyond a particular behaviour, fail to view the person as an individual, fail to view the behaviour as a form of communication or fail to understand the unmet need behind the behaviour (Kitwood, 1997). It is hard to provide an agreed definition for challenging behaviour because we all experience behaviour subjectively and have different expectations, skills and tolerance levels. A helpful broad definition is: '… the sorts of things that people do which others find unwelcome or even offensive' (Killick and Allan, 2001, p. 59).

As carers, the most fundamental skill we need is the ability to 'stand back' from a potentially difficult situation and consider the possible causes, meaning and responses to challenging behaviour through reflection. The question 'Who is this behaviour a problem for?' is a good starting-point. If an older person behaves in a way that is odd or surprising, an intervention is only indicated if the behaviour is distressing to the person or others, or if it results in unacceptable risk to the person or others. It is thought that as many as two-thirds of older people with dementia and behavioural disturbances are not distressed by their experiences (Ballard and Hulford, 2004). Consider the following example. Mrs Wright often responds to visual hallucinations of children by talking to them. She is not distressed by these experiences; in fact, she says she quite enjoys them. Although her family and carers find it a little hard to know how to react when she is talking to the 'children', the behaviour is not causing any particular distress or risk, and the most appropriate course of action is to monitor the situation.

How common is challenging behaviour in older people?

In a recent survey of registered mental health nurses in my Trust (from community, day hospital and ward teams), we ranked frequency of contact with challenging behaviour. We identified 22 behaviours which nurses viewed as 'challenging' and ranked these according to how frequently they were experienced during the course of our work. The results surprised us. We had been expecting aggression and violence to feature among the top three, but we discovered that the most commonly experienced behaviours were:

- repetitive speech;
- resisting care;
- repetitive actions;
- trying to leave/running away;
- screaming or shouting.

(McGeorge, 2005).

In a review of previous reports, Cohen-Mansfield and Taylor (1998) found the following variable prevalence rates among groups of older people with mental health conditions:

- pacing/wandering … 3–59%;
- noisy / disruptive vocal behaviour … 10–30%;
- aggressive behaviour … 8–49%.

Our local findings support other survey reports (Kovach et al., 2005), which indicate that aggression is not the most common form of challenging behaviour. However, other forms of behaviour are very common and experienced by an estimated 85% of all people with dementia at some time (Homefirst Community Trust, 2002).

Why is it important to learn about challenging behaviour?

Apart from the prevalence and likelihood that you will come across an older person with challenging behaviour at some point in your career, there are a number of other important reasons for learning more about challenging behaviour. The consequences for the person with 'behavioural disturbance' can include:

- increased use of chemical and physical restraints and the complications of these (Allen, 1999);
- increased likelihood of institutionalisation (Allen, 1999; Gerdner et al., 2002);
- increased care-giver stress (Gerdner et al., 2002) (including staff stress);
- increased unmet needs (Allen, 1999, Kovach et al., 2005);
- increased potential for carer abuse (Homer and Gilleard, 1990);
- adverse outcomes for family caregivers including depression and decline in physical health (Gerdner et al., 2002).

Understanding behavioural approaches and assessing behaviour

It is widely accepted that our behaviour is shaped by our personality, experiences, learning and the environment in the broadest sense (including physical and psychosocial aspects) (Wells and Wells, 1997). Behavioural therapy or behavioural modification focuses on changing behaviour through one or more of the following approaches:

- positive reinforcement – a pleasurable consequence of a behaviour, which increases the likelihood of the behaviour being repeated (e.g. being praised for an action);
- negative reinforcement – the ending of an unpleasant situation as a result of the behaviour, which increases the likelihood of the behaviour being repeated (e.g. relief from pain as a result of getting up and walking around);
- positive punishment – a disagreeable consequence following a behaviour, which reduces the likelihood of the behaviour being repeated;
- negative punishment – the removal of something pleasant as a consequence of a behaviour, which reduces the likelihood of the behaviour being repeated.

Positive reinforcement is the most common approach used with older people, and although there is a place for other behavioural modification techniques, such programmes should be used consciously, judiciously and as part of an agreed plan of treatment and care. Techniques requiring the ability to learn from the consequences of behaviour may not be suitable for all people with dementia, and most approaches demand consistent application with no variation between staff members. It is advisable to involve a team member with recognised specialist knowledge and skills before embarking on a behavioural-modification programme. Behaviour modification is often perceived as a reward-based approach to bringing about behavioural change. While its efficacy is widely recognised, there are those who perceive there to be ethical problems in trying to change the behaviour of a person with dementia through the use of rewards.

ABC charts

In order to reduce challenging behaviour or the risks it causes, we need to assess and record patterns of behaviour so that we can identify any underlying causes or triggers (McGonigal-Kenney and Schutte, 2006). An assessment which records not only details of the behaviour and its antecedents (triggers), but also the consequences, may help to identify any positive or negative reinforcers that maintain the behaviour. These assessments are sometimes referred to as ABC charts.

- A = antecedent, the catalyst or trigger for the behaviour,
- B = a description of the behaviour, what the person said or did; and
- C = consequences or reinforcer, or 'what happened next'.

For fairly discrete behavioural problems ABC charting may be required for only a very short period of time, and the act of recording the behaviour and circumstances may in itself be sufficient to understand any triggers or reinforcers; for example I worked with an older female whom staff described as 'very agitated and aggressive'. We introduced an ABC chart, and staff completed it for 12 hours. It soon became apparent that her swearing and restlessness were an indication that she needed to urinate, and we were able to plan care that met her needs and reduced her distress. For more complex or less frequent behavioural problems, an ABC chart may need to be completed for a more prolonged period (see Wells and Wells, 1997, for more detail).

Table 13.1 shows an excerpt from a completed ABC chart.

Other tools and scales

There are numerous behavioural rating scales and tools that can be used to monitor and evaluate the severity of a patient's behavioural disturbance. Examples of these (e.g. the Brief Agitation Rating Scale (BARS) and the Disruptive Behaviour Rating Scales (DBRS)) can be found in Burns et al. (1999). You should be aware that some tools require training before use and others require the purchase of a licence.

Table 13.1 Excerpt from an ABC chart

Date	Time	Antecedent	Behaviour	Consequence	Initials
ABC chart for Mrs Jane Cook Ward 11					
11.04.06	06.10	Awoke early to use the toilet; on coming out of her bedroom she could not find her way and was approached by myself – I tried to direct her to the toilet.	Mrs Cook became abusive and swore at me, telling me to leave her house. She threatened me, with her fist.	I withdrew and allowed Mrs Cook to look around the ward. After a few minutes, I reminded her where the toilet was, and she used it.	SJM
11.04.06	13.35	In the ward lounge after lunch with several other patients. TV on.	NA Brown heard Mrs Cook shouting at another patient, calling him a 'dirty devil' and 'leave me alone you vile creature'.	NA Brown approached Mrs Cook, but she was very distressed and angry. After a few minutes, the situation calmed, and NA Brown was able to distract Mrs Cook by showing her a magazine.	PJ
14.04.06	13.55	Lunch was cleared away, and most staff were in handover. The lounge was quiet, with only two other patients.	Another patient sat in a chair by the window and Mrs Cook shouted at her to 'get out – I want to sit there, you little tart'.	I had to intervene, as it looked like Mrs Cook was going to tip the chair over to remove the other patient. Mrs Cook tried to strike me with her fist but missed. I called for help, and we persuaded Mrs Cook to sit in the quiet room with company from NA Dade.	BB

The importance of clear description and documentation

In a study, Bair et al. (1999) found that behavioural problems were documented less than 1% of the time in medical records. Broad generic terms such as 'agitation' are usually unhelpful. Consider the following entry from a patient's health record: 'Mrs Cook remained agitated throughout the shift.' Does this entry convey any useful information to the nurse reading it? Are you able to form a picture of the way in which Mrs Cook was behaving and the circumstances of her behaviour? We probably all have different understandings and interpretations of what 'agitation' is. In verbal and written communication with colleagues, it is important to be explicit and precise about the nature of the person's behaviour. For example, in this case, the nursing record might state:

'Mrs Cook was unable to sit still during breakfast for more than a couple of minutes. She kept getting up from the table and searching through her handbag. She returned to the table each time she was prompted. Later, she attended the current affairs discussion, but after several minutes she became talkative and frequently interrupted other people who were trying to speak. When asked to allow other people a turn, she became cross and left the group.'

This entry gives enough detail for the reader to understand what happened and the context of Mrs Cook's behaviour and allows them to assess any subsequent improvement or deterioration.

Causes of challenging behaviour

McMinn and Draper (2005) point out that the care styles and systems we operate may in fact contribute to the development or maintenance of challenging behaviour. They assert that numerous short nurse–patient interactions can contribute to overstimulation or be a powerful reinforcer of behaviour. In addition to this, failure to provide consistency of staffing through shift systems and use of casual staff can contribute to a lack of continuity.

Using an environmental-behaviour approach, Allen (1999) identifies the causes of challenging behaviour as:

- overstimulation;
- understimulation;
- misperceptions (due to sensory loss);
- new environments;
- poor communication.

The person-centred care approach considers behaviour to be a form of communication and encourages carers faced with problematic behaviour to reflect 'what is this person trying to tell me?' It asserts that challenging behaviour is a consequence of 'malignant social psychology'; this is discussed earlier in Chapters 1 and 4.

Table 13.2 Examples of 'triggers' or causes for challenging behaviour

Physical	• Pain, hunger, thirst, need to eliminate, breathing problems, inadequate sleep, lack of exercise, failure of communication, dehydration, infection, metabolic or endocrine disturbance
Psychological	• Inability to understand language or visual cues • Hallucinations, delusions, illusions and misinterpretations • Failure of or inability to use usual coping strategies • Personality – possible exaggeration of previous traits • Anxiety and fear • Losses (of people, role and abilities,) • Illness-related problems, e.g. frontal-lobe dysfunction and cognitive impairment • Malignant social psychology
Social	• Lack of meaningful contact with others • Inadequate social-support mechanisms • Isolation • Group living • Change to usual routine • Malignant social psychology
Environmental	• Noise, poor lighting, intense lighting and environmental temperature • Lack of stimulation or too much stimulation • Lack of privacy • Unable to find way around, poor signs or visual cues • Routines designed around the needs of the organisation or staff rather than around the needs of older people

By combining these approaches, we can categorise triggers or causes of challenging behaviour into physical, psychological, social or environmental causes and models tend to focus on one or more of these areas. These are shown in Table 13.2.

Models seek to help us to understand why a person behaves or responds in a certain way and also to identify what we can do to reduce behaviour that causes a problem to the person or others. Challenging-behaviour models each have a different emphasis: some regard behaviour as an expression of need or unmet need (e.g. NDB); some regard behaviour as a consequence of environmental influences (e.g. Progressively Lowered Stress Threshold model; Smith and Buckwalter, 2005), and others regard behaviour as communication (e.g. person-centred care approaches). These approaches have many things in common and are not necessarily mutually exclusive.

Example of a model in action

The NDB proposes that 'background factors' (e.g. neurological, cognitive, health state and psychosocial history) and 'proximal factors' (physiological needs, psychological needs and physical and social environments) interact to produce need-driven behaviours (Whall and Kolanowski, 2004). By manipulating proximal factors that are associated with a particular behaviour (e.g. environmental noise), the individual may be helped to meet their own needs. This model was used to help plan care for the following older person. Mr Fisher (79 years old) is a patient on an acute medical ward. He was admitted with shortness of breath and mild confusion and is known to have vascular dementia. He is currently being treated for heart failure and is being nursed in a single room because of an infection. He was referred to the mental health liaison nurse on day 7 of his admission because of 'behavioural problems'. Nurses on the ward say that he constantly shouts but that when they attend him, he either makes very minor requests (e.g. 'pass me my drink') or cannot tell them what he wanted. Figure 13.1 demonstrates how this model was applied.

While we may not be able to change or impact on the 'background' factors, carers may be in a position to modify the 'proximal' factors. When Mr Fisher's

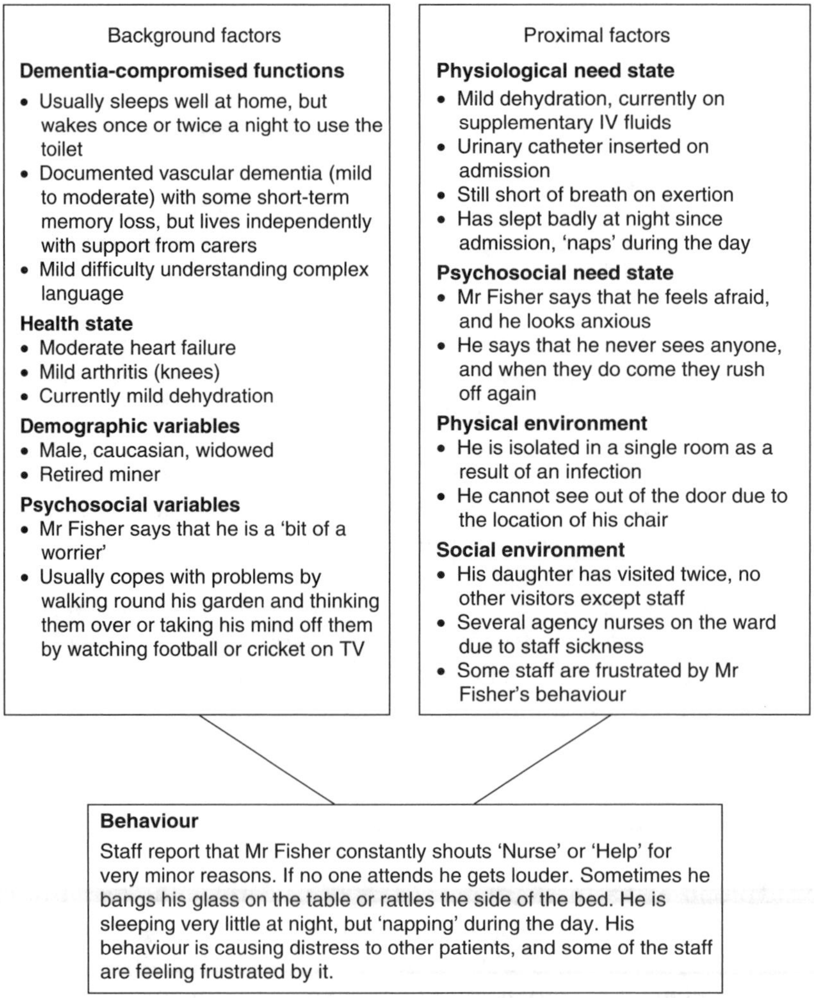

Background factors

Dementia-compromised functions
- Usually sleeps well at home, but wakes once or twice a night to use the toilet
- Documented vascular dementia (mild to moderate) with some short-term memory loss, but lives independently with support from carers
- Mild difficulty understanding complex language

Health state
- Moderate heart failure
- Mild arthritis (knees)
- Currently mild dehydration

Demographic variables
- Male, caucasian, widowed
- Retired miner

Psychosocial variables
- Mr Fisher says that he is a 'bit of a worrier'
- Usually copes with problems by walking round his garden and thinking them over or taking his mind off them by watching football or cricket on TV

Proximal factors

Physiological need state
- Mild dehydration, currently on supplementary IV fluids
- Urinary catheter inserted on admission
- Still short of breath on exertion
- Has slept badly at night since admission, 'naps' during the day

Psychosocial need state
- Mr Fisher says that he feels afraid, and he looks anxious
- He says that he never sees anyone, and when they do come they rush off again

Physical environment
- He is isolated in a single room as a result of an infection
- He cannot see out of the door due to the location of his chair

Social environment
- His daughter has visited twice, no other visitors except staff
- Several agency nurses on the ward due to staff sickness
- Some staff are frustrated by Mr Fisher's behaviour

Behaviour

Staff report that Mr Fisher constantly shouts 'Nurse' or 'Help' for very minor reasons. If no one attends he gets louder. Sometimes he bangs his glass on the table or rattles the side of the bed. He is sleeping very little at night, but 'napping' during the day. His behaviour is causing distress to other patients, and some of the staff are feeling frustrated by it.

Fig. 13.1   Example of application of the need-driven dementia-compromised behaviour model.

assessment was completed using the NDB model, the mental-health liaison nurse was able to help the ward team consider what might be contributing to his behaviour, and they identified the following possibilities.

Factors which may be contributing to Mr Fisher's 'calling out':

- isolation from others in the single room; he can't see anyone else;
- infrequent and short visits from staff;
- few visits from family or friends; he could be lonely;
- he may be anxious about what is happening to him or because he is still breathless;
- lack of restful sleep;
- poor short-term memory, which means that he cannot remember when he last saw someone;
- nothing to occupy his mind; no TV or radio in the room;
- some staff feel frustrated with Mr Fisher; it may affect the way they communicate with him, and he may recognise this.

It also seemed possible that the frequent short visits from staff were positively reinforcing Mr Fisher's calling out, thus perpetuating the behaviour. As a result of greater understanding, the ward team successfully implemented a plan of care that involved:

- twice daily more prolonged contact with a staff member (at least 30 minutes), even when there was no physical care to be provided;
- a member of the team 'looking in' on Mr Fisher every 10 minutes throughout the day and night and asking him whether he needed anything (gradually the frequency was extended to every 30 minutes);
- provision of a TV so that Mr Fisher could watch sports programmes when he wanted to.

Mr Fisher's shouting decreased from the first day the plan was implemented, although there were still times when he would shout in between visits from staff. As his physical condition improved, he was moved to a bay with other patients, and the shouting almost completely resolved.

The principle underlying the approach used with Mr Fisher was to remove or manipulate triggers or causes of his behaviour in order to reduce it or prevent it from happening. Some authors refer to this as 'anticipatory care', which is: 'actions taken before the usual time of onset of a particular problem in order to prevent or moderate the occurrence of the problem.' (Kovach et al., 2005, p. 138)

The outcome of anticipatory care is a reduction in unmet needs, thereby reducing the likelihood and incidence of challenging behaviour and enhancing the quality of life for the older person.

Interventions for older people with challenging behaviour

Because of our individuality, there is no 'one size fits all' answer to reducing challenging behaviour. What works in one situation may not work again with another person. Unfortunately, there is no 'magic' or easy solution to alleviating challenging behaviour; it is a complex task. Developing an understanding of the person and finding solutions that work for them takes considerable effort, perseverance and cooperation from the whole team. Often, several potential solutions will need to be tried out in practice and their effects closely observed. Maintaining a consistent approach from all members of the team as well as motivation are further challenges and an important role for the primary nurse, named nurse or care coordinator.

James et al. (2004) divide possible interventions into two categories; general (or 'non-specific') and problem-focused. They believe that interventions in the first group are aimed at promoting positive well-being and tend to focus on a person's strengths, supporting the person in difficulty and fostering psychological well-being through validation of experiences. This group of interventions includes reality orientation, validation techniques, reminiscence therapy, art, music and activity, complementary therapy and multi-sensory approaches. The evidence of effectiveness for these interventions is not robust and there are strong recommendations for further research (Neal and Briggs 2003; Woods et al., 2005), but there is often experiential and anecdotal evidence of the acceptability and benefit of these interventions on an individual basis. The problem-focused group of interventions includes behaviour therapy or modification, cognitive behaviour therapy and interpersonal therapy (James et al., 2004), for which there is better evidence of effectiveness.

Non-pharmacological interventions should be used as the first-choice treatment for behavioural problems (National Institute for Clinical Excellence, 2006), and medication should be used as a last resort and then reserved for people with the most challenging or risky behaviour. There is little robust evidence that medication is effective in reducing challenging behaviour and potentially harmful side effects are well recognised (e.g. sedation, extra-pyramidal effects, falls, reduced quality of life and accelerated cognitive decline) (Ballard and Hulford, 2004). Some of the drugs used (e.g. anti-psychotics) can increase agitation, but, despite this, there is still widespread use of neuroleptic medication, especially in institutional care.

Simple first steps when caring for a patient with challenging behaviour are likely to happen concurrently rather than in a linear manner:

- establish effective communication; this includes knowledge of the person;
- maximise sensory perception (e.g. by ensuring the person's hearing aid works and they are wearing it or by reducing background noise);
- build a relationship based on trust and rapport;
- ask the person and/or carers what they think is the cause of the behaviour, and what they think might help or how they have coped with it in the past;
- assess the person and environment for risks and reduce any risks that may be caused by the person's behaviour;
- observe, record and interpret the person's behaviour – consider using the ABC approach;

- adopt a systematic 'trial and error' approach to altering triggers/stimuli/the environment;
- evaluate the impact of 'trials' to reduce challenging behaviour;
- document and communicate your evaluation with the team, the older person and carers.

Caring for people who resist essential care

There is limited literature and evidence outlining effective interventions in caring for older people who resist care. Werner et al. (2002) consider that this type of behaviour relates to withstanding or opposing the efforts of a caregiver. Situations involving resistance can manifest in a variety of ways, for example, pushing the caregiver away, hitting, nipping, lack of cooperation, refusing to stand up to have clothing put on, screaming or shouting. A variety of triggers have been identified, which may result in screaming and shouting. These include sensory deprivation, discomfort or pain, fatigue, over- or understimulation, or noise (Sloane and Barrick, 1998). Buhr and White (2006) suggest that music, simulated presence therapy or multi-sensory techniques may help calm the person when shouting or screaming. Furthermore, they suggest the following strategies to assist with resistance:

- Use reasoning and distraction.
- Promote the patient's independence and autonomy.
- Create a predictable routine, approach the person from the front and maintain eye contact, explain what will be happening, allow participation in Activities of Daily Living, ensure privacy during personal care tasks and postpone the activity if needed (Buhr and White, 2006).

While these strategies have a role to play, it is also worth considering that some people with dementia will have 'favourite carers'. It may be that they will respond in a more receptive way to some people and, while this may not always be achievable or desirable, it is worthy of consideration.

Caring for under-active or passive people

In a study set on a Geriatric Evaluation Unit in a large teaching hospital, Bair et al. (1999) found that hypo-active physical disruptive behaviours occurred almost as frequently as hyper-active physical and verbal behaviours, but were much less frequently recognised by care staff. The study found that nurses tend to focus on people with overt behaviour, e.g. aggression or shouting rather than those who were passive and less likely to attract attention. Colling (2004) offers useful advice for dealing with the passive individual, which includes giving cues and assistance, initiating tasks and giving guidance to allow the older person to participate and enjoy activities.

Caring for older people who may be aggressive

Although nurses often focus upon those individuals who are shouting or being aggressive, these types of situations are not always handled well by health professionals. In older people with dementia, aggression is frequently associated with intrusions into their personal space, particularly by carers (Cohen-Mansfield and Taylor, 1998). Physical interventions such as Control and Restraint techniques can be potentially harmful to older people and should only be used under expert guidance. Some providers of care offer training in the use of specific techniques that are safer to use with older people, but use of these should always be a last resort. Chapter 7 discusses restraint in more detail.

Caring for people with hallucinations

Asking the question 'who is the hallucination a problem for?' is a good starting-point when caring for someone experiencing hallucinations. Some older people who hallucinate do not find it distressing or unpleasant. Deciding how to respond to a person who is hallucinating depends upon knowledge and assessment of the situation. Some older people recognise that they are hallucinating and may be reassured by explanations of what is happening to them. Other people may not be aware that they are hallucinating and may be insistent that what they see or hear is really happening. In such situations, it is best not to argue with the person; there may even be times when it is most effective to 'go along' with the hallucination; for example, a carer told me that every night she had to order her husband's 'visitors' to leave the house before he would go upstairs to bed. Distraction, conversation, company and activity can all help to reduce distress caused by hallucinations. The Alzheimer's Society (2000) advice sheet 'Hallucinations and Delusions' provides further useful information.

Caring for people with delusions

Delusional thinking can present as suspiciousness or paranoia in older people, and this may be manifested in unusual behaviour; for example, an older lady who put her food in her pockets and handbag and threw it out of the window later disclosed that she did so because she believed someone had 'tampered with it'. Changing the focus of the person's attention away from the delusions can be helpful. Arguing or disputing the person's beliefs is usually counterproductive and may result in the person believing that you are also 'against' them.

Recognising and validating the person's feelings may also be useful. For example, I could respond to an older man telling me that he is being poisoned by saying 'You must be feeling very alone and frightened'. However, identifying things that make the person feel 'safe' must be an individualised task, as any error may make the situation worse.

Caring for older people who 'wander' or 'pace'

Triggers which may result in wandering or pacing may include insecurity or disorientation to a new environment, a feeling of loss, excess energy, pain or discomfort, boredom, maintenance of usual routines, elimination problems, noise or drug-induced restlessness (Brennan, 1999). Buhr and White (2006) suggest that encouraging exercise, providing a safe and pleasant place to walk and providing structured individualised activities may all help to minimise pacing or wandering. Dewing (2005) offers a useful screening tool which can be easily used by nurses.

Conclusion

Providing care for older people with behaviours that challenge is a complex but often rewarding role. It requires careful and sometimes detailed assessment, development and delivery of individualised plans of care, a systematic 'trial-and-error' approach to the use of a range of interventions and evaluation of their effectiveness. Through identifying the causes of a particular behaviour, we may be able to manipulate the environment, our own response or the response of others to alleviate the older person's distress, thus reducing challenging behaviour and improving their quality of life. Finally, general principles for working with older people who have challenging behaviour are summarised in Box 13.1.

Box 13.1   General principles for working with older people who have challenging behaviour

- **Attitude:** relaxed, flexible, smiling caregivers, humour, patience and maintaining a quiet and calm environment.
- **Empathy:** recognition that behavioural problems can cause fear, distress and avoidance in caregivers (Woods et al., 2004).
- **Positive communication:** responses that hinder (and so should be avoided) include 'correcting', putting stress on the person, rushing activities and repeating directions, demonstrating frustration or irritation (Colling, 2004). Avoid accentuating a person's mistakes and failings, instead, emphasise their strengths and achievements (Buijssen, 2005). Say positive things about the person, use distraction and redirection, and avoid arguing (Buhr and White 2006).
- **Involving carers:** and maintaining contact with family and friends were identified as positive approaches (Colling, 2004).
- A range of **therapeutic approaches** should be available to older people because it is impossible to predict which intervention will prove effective in which situation. Approaches include distraction, redirection, validation, diversion, occupation/activity, sensory techniques, reminiscence, reality orientation and music therapy.
- **Sensitive communication:** using the person's preferred form of address, a calm, quiet approach, a level of language, which the person is most likely to understand (e.g. simple one-stage commands rather than complex instructions), use of non-verbal communication, sensitive use of personal space and touch.

Box 13.1   (Continued)

- **Self-awareness:** the conscious recognition of how a person or a situation is making you feel, and how this might affect your reactions and the ability to withhold from the person feelings of irritation, frustration, failure, etc.
- The ability to contribute to and communicate an **assessment** of the person's behaviour, through observation and accurate reporting.
- The ability to 'listen' to the person's behaviour and assist in **interpreting** what might be triggers and alleviating factors.
- **Monitoring** and **evaluation** of interventions as they are put into practice.
- **Manipulating the environment** to meet the needs of individual people can be difficult where a group of people have diverse needs, and compromises may have to be made. The 'environment' includes routine and structure to the day, and levels of activity and stimulation that meet the needs of the person.
- Use of **positive reinforcement** to encourage desired behaviour.
- Effective utilisation of **reflection** and **clinical supervision** is crucial to the development and maintenance of effective skills.

References

Allen, L.A. (1999) Treating agitation without drugs. *American Journal of Nursing* **99** (4), 36–42.

Alzheimer's Society (2000) *Hallucinations and Delusions: Advice Sheet*. London, Alzheimer's Society.

Bair, B., Toth, W., Johnson, M.A., Rosenberg, C. and Hurdle, J.F. (1999) Interventions for disruptive behaviours: use and success. *Journal of Gerontological Nursing* **25** (1), 13–20.

Ballard, C. and Hulford, L. (2004) Drugs used to relieve behavioural symptoms of dementia. *Nursing and Residential Care* **6** (7), 342–346.

Brennan, S. (1999) Wandering and restraint: the carer's dilemma. *Nursing and Residential Care* **1** (1), 14–19.

Buhr, G.T. and White, H.K. (2006) Difficult behaviors in long-term care patients with dementia. *Journal of the American Medical Directors Association* **7**, 180–192.

Buijssen, H. (2005) *The Simplicity of Dementia. A Guide for Family and Carers*. London, Jessica Kingsley.

Burns, A., Lawlor, B. and Craig, S. (1999) *Assessment Scales in Old Age Psychiatry*. London, Martin Dunitz.

Chiu, E. (1991) Psychiatric disorders in later life. In: *The Challenge of Ageing: a Multidisciplinary Approach to Extended Care* (M.W. Shaw, ed.). Melbourne, Churchill Livingstone, pp. 113–119.

Cohen-Mansfield, J. and Taylor, L. (1998) Assessing and understanding agitated behaviours in older adults. In: *Behaviours in Dementia: Best Practices for Successful Management* (M. Kaplan and S.B. Hoffman, eds). Baltimore, MD, Health Professions, pp. 25–44.

Colling, K.B. (2004) Caregiver interventions for passive behaviors in dementia: links to the NDB model. *Aging and Mental Health* **8** (2), 117–125.

Dewing, J. (2005) Screening for wandering among older persons with dementia. *Nursing Older People* **17** (3), 20–24.

Gerdner, L.A., Buckwalter, K.C. and Reed, D. (2002) Impact of a psychoeducational intervention on caregiver response to behavioural problems. *Nursing Research* **51** (6), 363–374.

Homefirst Community Trust (2002) *Coping with Maggie – Caring for Margaret. Communicating through Behaviour: A Person Centred Approach to Caring for People with Dementia*. Ballymena, UK, Homefirst Community Trust.

Homer, A.C. and Gilleard, C. (1990) Abuse of elderly people by their carers. *British Medical Journal* **301**, 1359–1362.

James, I., Douglas, S. and Ballard, C. (2004) Different forms of psychological interventions in dementia. *Nursing and Residential Care* **6** (6), 288–291.

Killick, J. and Allan, K. (2001) *Communication and the Care of People with Dementia*. Buckingham, UK, Open University Press.

Kitwood, T. (1997) *Dementia Reconsidered: The Person Comes First*. Buckingham, UK, Open University Press.

Kovach, C.R., Noonan, P.E., Schildt, A.M. and Wells, T. (2005) A model of consequences of need-driven dementia-compromised behaviour. *Journal of Nursing Scholarship* **37** (2), 134–140.

McGeorge, S. (2005) *Mental Health Services for Older People: Challenging Behaviour Survey Results*. Unpublished. County Durham and Darlington Priority Services NHS Trust.

McGonigal-Kenney, M.L. and Schutte, D.L. (2006) Evidence-based guideline: nonpharmacologic management of agitated behaviors in persons with Alzheimer Disease and other chronic dementing conditions. *Journal of Gerontological Nursing* **32** (2), 9–14.

McMinn, B. and Draper, B. (2005) Vocally disruptive behaviour in dementia: development of an evidence based practice guideline. *Aging and Mental Health* **9** (1), 16–24.

Neal, M. and Barton Wright, P. Validation therapy for dementia. *The Cochrane Database of Systematic Reviews 2003,* Issue 3. Art. No.: CD001394. DOI: 10.1002/14651858. CD001394.

National Institute for Clinical Excellence (2006) Dementia: Supporting People with Dementia and their Carers. Draft Guideline, May 2006. http://www.nice.org.uk/page.aspx?o=315284

Sloane, P.D. and Barrick, A.L. (1998) Management of occasional and frequent problem behaviours in dementia. In: *Behaviours in Dementia: Best Practices for Successful Management* (M. Kaplan and S.B. Hoffman, eds), Baltimore, MD, Health Professions Press.

Smith, M. and Buckwalter, K. (2005) Behaviors associated with dementia. *American Journal of Nursing* **105** (7), 40–52.

Wells, C. and Wells, J. (1997) Reducing challenging behaviour of elderly confused people: a behavioural perspective. In: *Mental Health Care for Elderly People* (I.J. Norman and S.J. Redfern, eds). New York, Churchill Livingstone.

Werner, P., Tabak, N., Alpert, R. and Bergman, R. (2002) Interventions used by nursing staff members with psychogeriatric patients resisting care. *International Journal of Nursing Studies* **39**, 461–467.

Whall, A.L. and Kolanowski, A.M. (2004) Editorial: the need-driven dementia-compromised behaviour model – a framework for understanding the behavioural symptoms of dementia. *Aging and Mental Health* **8** (2), 106–108.

Woods, B., Spector, A., Jones, C., Orrell, M. and Davies, S. Reminiscence therapy for dementia. *The Cochrane Database of Systematic Reviews 2005*, Issue 2. Art. No.: CD001120. DOI: 10.1002/14651858. CD001120.pub2.

Woods, D.L., Rapp, C.G. and Beck, C. (2004) Escalation/de-escalation patterns of behavioural symptoms of persons with dementia. *Aging and Mental Health* **8** (2), 126–132.

Chapter 14
Delirium

Irene Schofield

Introduction

Delirium or acute confusion is a syndrome (cluster of symptoms) which occurs as a sudden and fluctuating impairment in mental status secondary to a medical condition or its treatment. Older adults are thought to be at risk of developing delirium concurrent with acute illness as a result of physical ageing processes, in particular those which affect neurotransmitter function in the brain. Delirium often presents as the major feature of a life-threatening condition or as a serious complication of illness in an older person. It is often the first and only sign of pneumonia, sepsis and myocardial infarction. It is vital, therefore, that nurses are skilled in its detection.

There are many studies and descriptive articles in the medical and nursing literature on the incidence, causes and care of patients with delirium; there are very few, however, which address the experience of the older person with delirium. This omission serves to minimise the significance of delirium to the individual concerned. This chapter will draw on empirical evidence, expert clinical experience from the seminal work of the USA psychiatrist Lipowski and doctoral research in progress. These will raise awareness of the effects of delirium on the person who experiences it. The overall chapter aim is to highlight the knowledge and skills required to be proactive and supportive in caring for an older person who develops delirium.

It is important, first of all, to clarify the use of terminology with regard to 'delirium' and 'acute confusion' because although 'delirium' is the term used by international disease classification systems, it is still not widely understood and used in clinical practice. Nurses, for example, use 'confusion' or 'acute confusion', while doctors use 'delirium' to describe the same phenomenon (Milisen et al., 2002). Nurses commonly use the generic term 'confusion' to describe cognition and behaviour that differs from a person's usual state and as an imprecise substitute for the many different features of mental impairment (Lipowski, 1990). 'Confusion' is often used incorrectly as a diagnosis rather than as a complex symptom with many different features.

Delirium is most often a transient and reversible cause of mental impairment (see Box 14.1 for the full definition).

Box 14.1 Definition of delirium

Delirium is characterised by a disturbance of consciousness and a change in cognition that develop over a short period of time. The disorder has a tendency to fluctuate during the course of the day, and there is evidence from the history, examination or investigations that the delirium is a direct consequence of a general medical condition

In order to make a diagnosis of delirium, a patient must show each of the features 1–4 listed below:

(1) Disturbance of consciousness (i.e. reduced clarity of awareness of the environment) with reduced ability to focus, sustain or shift attention.

(2) A change in cognition (such as memory deficit, disorientation, language disturbance) or the development of a perceptual disturbance that is not better accounted for by a pre-existing or evolving dementia.

(3) The disturbance developing over a short period of time (usually hours to days) and tending to fluctuate during the course of the day.

(4) Evidence from the history, physical examination or laboratory tests that the disturbance is caused by the direct physiological consequences of a general medical condition, substance intoxication or withdrawal, use of a medication, toxin exposure or a combination of these factors (American Psychiatric Association, 1994, p. 123).

Although older people in any setting can present with delirium concurrent with the development of a medical condition or its treatment, it is mostly studied and described in hospital patients. It is suggested that in general hospitals, 20% of older patients (range 7–61%) will develop delirium, and in patients who undergo surgery for fractured neck of femur prevalence varies between 10 and 50% (British Geriatrics Society, 2005). Delirium is often not recognised, and its effect on the well-being, future care and survival of the older person is underestimated. The consequences of a person developing delirium, however, have been widely studied. A diagnosis of delirium can interfere with a person's understanding of, and participation in, treatment and therapy, resulting in a slower rate of recovery and prolonged time in hospital (Faculty of Old Age Psychiatry, 2005). Delirium is associated with unwanted consequences such as falls, fractures, the development of pressure ulcers and patients pulling at or removing their own catheters and drainage tubes. It may interfere with nutrition, hydration and the administration of medicines. Morbidity and mortality are increased, and a hospital patient is more likely to be discharged to a care home (Faculty of Old Age Psychiatry, 2005).

Full recovery is the most common outcome for delirium, and this is influenced by age, morbidity, underlying causes, appropriateness, effectiveness and timeliness of treatment and support. It is usual to recover from delirium within a week, but there is increasing evidence to suggest that delirious episodes may recur for several weeks, or months, especially at night (Faculty of Old Age Psychiatry, 2005). Delirium is, therefore, a serious threat to the continuing independence of older people, and early detection and appropriate treatment have been shown to improve outcomes for older people with delirium and delirium superimposed on dementia (Cole, 2004).

Risk factors for developing delirium

Many studies have identified different risk factors for delirium. The complex profile of multiple pathology, however, in hospitalised older people complicates the task of identifying single risk factors, and a multifactoral cause is thought to be the most common. In the case of a person undergoing surgery, for example, delirium may be precipitated by intra- or post-operative hypotension, intra- or post-operative hypothermia, haemorrhage, hypoxia, imposed immobilisation, sensory overload, sleep deprivation and the anticholinergic effects of medications such as anaesthetics, analgesics and anti-emetics.

One theory towards risk of developing delirium is that predisposing factors interact with precipitating factors. Predisposing factors are present at the time of hospital admission and reflect the person's essential vulnerability, while precipitating factors are those additional factors which contribute to the development of delirium (Inouye, 1999). When Inouye and colleagues analysed the precipitating factors and previously identified predisposing factors, delirium rates increased progressively from low-risk to high-risk groups. They concluded that precipitating and predisposing factors are highly interrelated and contribute to delirium both independently and cumulatively. In addition, clinical judgement plays an important role in recognising the interplay between the two as a means of identifying high-risk patients (Inouye and Charpentier, 1996). For example, a patient with high vulnerability such as a pre-existing diagnosis of dementia, hearing impairment and vision impairment might develop delirium after receiving a single dose of night sedation. However, it could take major surgery such as a heart bypass operation and a stay in ITU to cause a fit, 80-year-old with no previous cognitive deficits to develop delirium.

Table 14.1 shows the risk factors for developing delirium, and Table 14.2 shows the precipitating factors for delirium.

Table 14.1   Predisposing factors for developing delirium

Older age
Severe illness
Dementia
Physical frailty
Admission with infection or dehydration
Visual impairment
Polypharmacy
Surgery e.g. fracture neck of femur
Alcohol excess
Renal impairment

British Geriatrics Society, (2005)

Table 14.2   Precipitating factors for delirium

Immobility
Use of physical restraint
Use of bladder catheter
Iatrogenic events
Malnutrition
Psychoactive medications
Intercurrent illness
Dehydration

British Geriatrics Society, (2005)

The experience of delirium

It has been suggested that confusion continues to be conceptualised and opera-
tionalised from an 'outsiders' perspective', so that the focus is on how confusion impacts on nurses and other patients rather than how it affects the person
themselves (Foreman, 1990). Foreman argues that the focus on the professional
view serves to limit our understanding of this phenomenon. Some understanding of the confused person's 'world' of delirium can help nurses to appreciate
the kinds of thoughts, feelings and perceptions that lie behind the behaviours
of confused patients.

In the hyperactive subtype, the person is visibly restless, excitable and on their
guard. They can be continuously on the move, searching, shouting, combative,
leaving their bed or ward and resisting when staff try to calm them. Perceptual
disorders such as illusions (based on fact and representing a misinterpretation
of the environment) and hallucinations (occur without any external stimulus)
are common, although they are not always present. Illusions are triggered by
darkness, shadows, sounds, and unfamiliarity of the setting. Visual hallucinations are the most common and are projected into nearby space. These are
often three-dimensional, moving, bright and coloured images of people or non-
human objects. Patients may be amused, be angry, appear detached or panic and
feel they need to get away from these objects (Lipowski, 1990; Schofield, 1997).
Anne Gould (an orthopaedic patient) in Case Study 14.1, however, seemed quite
unfazed by the cat and its interaction with the older woman.

Case study 14.1

'And the funniest thing, I saw an enormous Persian cat, now can you imagine a cat in a
hospital? I think it was the most beautiful thing I've ever seen. Then an elderly lady came
in and she started kissing this cat on its mouth. Now she's kissing and you know making
love to a male … But it was that cat across there, I swear if I'd see it I would know him
immediately, that cat'. (Schofield, 1997 p.945)

Lipowski (1990) speculates on the effect of delirium on an individual's emotions and mood. He suggests that emotional disturbances may reflect the

individual's personality, awareness and concern at being ill and cognitively impaired. According to Lipowski (1990), unconscious conflicts as well as guilt over actual or imagined wrongdoings may influence the content of hallucinations and the person's emotional and behavioural response to them. When delusions (false beliefs) occur in the context of suspicion and mistrust, such as when a patient believes that a nurse is poisoning them or keeping them captive, they may use atypically crude or sexually explicit language in defending their position. Lipowski (ibid.) observed that illusions can combine with intrusive powerful delusions as in the scenarios of Alfred Brown and Denis White. Alfred Brown in Case Study 14.2 was a patient in an acute medical ward. The hospital refuse collection took place in the early hours of the morning in the yard below the ward, and this may have been a trigger for Mr Brown's experiences.

Case study 14.2

'There was a raid – loads of lorries coming in and dashing about … outside there seemed a lot of soldiers there. One of them says, "I'm the Lieutenant Colonel." There was a lot of arguing amongst themselves and all of a sudden it finished. What has come to me is that this Lieutenant Colonel was a patient in here. He was up on a charge of falsifying accounts and he was found not guilty. And they were celebrating in here'. (Schofield, 1997, p .946)

Dennis White (a surgical patient) in Case Study 14.3 occupied a bed at the entrance to a surgical ward, and patients would be wheeled past him on trolleys when they were admitted to the ward and on their way to and from the operating theatre. He told me that he felt abandoned by his friends and that he was left to eat his meals on his own.

Case study 14.3

'I'd lie in bed and I'd see different forms and that in front of me. People … just come to you and look and grin and I used to ask them to help me get up and do things but they just stood there and grinned you know … like a big funeral I saw and it used to pass and the mourners used to go and it used to last all day long you know … you'd see them coming back from the funeral and that was coffin after coffin, coffin after coffin you know. Why it was I don't know'. (Schofield, 1997, p. 946)

Lipowski has suggested that the images which feature in illusions and hallucinations reflect the patient's current concerns and are often accompanied by intense emotions such as fear and anger. These may be linked to a recent or remote traumatic event. In their delirious state, the patient may find it difficult to separate fact from fantasy and dream from waking imagery, so it is as if they are experiencing them in tandem as in the case of James Green (an orthopaedic patient) in Case Study 14.4, whose delirium was most probably caused in part by post-operative pain (Schofield, 1997). He had dozed off in the evening and woke up suddenly with pain in his knee.

Case study 14.4

'I looked all round saw the television on all the lights were on, I said what the dickens is this, tried to get up and turn the telly off and couldn't get up. All the movements going on of the nurses and people talking, although I knew I was in a ward, I thought I was in my flat … I said the tablets were on the sideboard and just pointed … Things come to mind. I shouted, "nurse, nurse" and I just realised I was in hospital … because she came. I do dream a lot at home you know … but not a dream like this you know … vivid dream, so vivid it was, so vivid you know'. (Schofield, 1997, p. 946)

The hyperactive form of delirium frequently occurs as a critical situation in hospital at night, when the person who develops delirium is at risk of hurting themselves or others. A person in this situation can injure themselves as a result of tearing open sutures, pulling at intravenous lines or drainage tubes, or falling, and sustaining a fracture and/or head injury. A person who is fearful and mobile may feel an urgent need to flee the ward, oblivious to the danger that this might pose. The patients may eventually collapse if they are not calmed or sedated (Lipowski, 1990). It has been suggested that ward staff may equate delirium exclusively with this particular subtype, as patients with agitation are most likely to come to their attention (Lipowski, 1990; O'Keeffe and Lavan, 1997). Medication toxicity and withdrawal from medications and alcohol are particularly associated with the hyperactive-hyper alert subtype. Patients with the hyperactive-hyper alert form of delirium appear to have the highest rate of full recovery (O'Keeffe and Lavan, 1997).

In contrast, in the hypoactive subtype, the person is less physically active and alert than usual, responses and movements are slow and speech is hesitant. They are quiet and listless, and easily drift off to sleep during care or they lie with eyes open, seemingly indifferent to what is happening in their immediate surroundings (Lipowski, 1990). Although the patient may seem apathetic, lethargic and disconnected from their surroundings, they may experience distress and may hear what is being said about them. Vera Jones (a medical patient) describes her experience in Case Study 14.5.

Case study 14.5

'I don't remember coming in. I just found myself in. They tell me I was ill and needed to come in. I must have been in for a few days before I eventually came round to myself. I didn't know where I was … I was eating … They were looking after me. Apart from that I just didn't know where I was'. (Schofield, 1997, p 948)

It is important to assess whether the patient is easily distracted, or has difficulty switching attention from one topic to another and has difficulty keeping track of what you say. Persons with the hypoactive subtype are less able than usual to take cues from their surroundings in order to make sense of their environment. A person may be capable of responding to a simple greeting or brief questions with the result that this subtle presentation of delirium goes unrecognised in a busy ward. O'Keeffe and Lavan (1997) have suggested that infection and metabolic imbalance are the most likely causes of the hypoactive-hypoalert subtype. It may also mimic depression, in that patients appear withdrawn and slow in speech and movement, and experience sleep disturbances. A person's lack of attention or short attention span is central to the current definition of delirium, however, and would suggest a definitive diagnosis of delirium. The hypoactive or 'quiet' form of delirium is believed to be more common in people with dementia (Johnson, 1999), making it less likely to be recognised by medical and nursing staff, and therefore overlooked.

A combination of the above two clinical subtypes, known as the mixed type is most common (O'Keeffe, 1999). The person alternates unpredictably between the two types, during the course of a day or a few days. For all the subtypes, lucid intervals may occur, lasting minutes or hours, and these are most frequent during the day. Towards the evening and in the night, however, the disturbed and confused state returns. Disturbance of consciousness spans a spectrum of states from alertness to coma. Memory impairment is an integral feature of delirium. Orientation can be impaired with disorientation to time first to appear and last to disappear. This can be followed by disorientation to place, name and location. An ability to think clearly is crucial to feelings of security and self-esteem, and the sense of helplessness brought about by loss of intellectual and perceptual ability can be highly threatening and stressful. Feelings of paranoia are exacerbated by awareness of not being in control, feelings of helplessness and a need to be dependent on others. No two patients with the syndrome present the same clinical profile, and this hinders the recognition and study of delirium (Sandberg et al., 1999).

Identifying delirium

An important assessment challenge for staff is to be able to separate the new symptoms of delirium from any pre-existing symptoms of dementia so that delirium in a person with dementia is quickly identified, as it may be the only clue that they have a treatable medical condition. Obtaining information from relatives, neighbours or carers on the patient's usual mental functioning in order to detect changes is central to differentiating delirium from other types of mental impairment.

There are a number of screening tools to detect delirium, although many are not suitable for daily clinical use, as they are too long and complex. The tools presented here have been developed for routine clinical use by nurses. An ideal tool maintains psychometric rigour, differentiates delirium from other cognitive disorders, requires minimum training in its use, takes little staff time and is acceptable to patients. The latter is especially important in the detection of delirium because of the fluctuating nature of the condition. The more frequent the measurements, therefore, the greater the intrusion and increased stress for the older person. An effective instrument provides information on the progression of the condition and whether patients are responding to interventions and treatment.

A brief informal method of assessing attention/inattention is by asking the individual to recite the months of the year backwards or count backwards from 20 to 1. It is highly unlikely that a person with delirium will be able to achieve this. A widely used formal screening tool for delirium is the Confusion Assessment Method (CAM) (Inouye et al., 1990). It provides a sound basis for clinical decision-making and articulation of the presenting problems to a medical or senior nursing colleague. It takes the form of nine reflective questions which require some interpretation followed by an algorithm based on the central features of delirium. The CAM is easy to use and puts little pressure on patients and staff. It takes less than 5 minutes to complete. The CAM is limited, however, in that it does not measure the severity of an episode of delirium.

The NEECHAM Confusion Scale consists of nine components covering information processing, performance and vital function items. It combines nursing assessment and brief interactions with patients in a hospital setting. Completion of the scale takes 10 minutes. It has good validity and reliability (Neelon et al., 1996).

Schuurmans and colleagues have recently developed the 13-item Delirium Observation Screening (DOS) Scale. It takes only a few minutes to complete, and a diagnosis of delirium can be made (delirious or not) based on the results of three consecutive shifts (Schuurmans et al., 2002).

Prevention and care

The following quote from the seminal textbook *Confusion Prevention and Care* conveys the importance of quickly getting to the root cause of confusion in order to maintain a person's respect and dignity: '. . . providing emergency treatment for confusion is similar to administering cardiopulmonary resuscitation; unless the underlying problem is identified and treated, the result is a kind of death, for socially the confused person becomes a nonperson' (Wolanin and Phillips, 1981).

Empirical studies

There is accumulating research evidence to demonstrate that delirium is preventable in up to one-third of patients (Inouye et al., 1999) by anticipating its occurrence and manipulating the modifiable risk factors discussed previously. Interventions that have been demonstrated to be effective in preventing or decreasing the severity of delirium include effective interpersonal communication, environmental modification, consultations with specialist medical and nursing teams and specific actions to eliminate known modifiable risk factors. Many studies, however, test a combination of interventions, so that it is sometimes impossible to say which ones had the most effect. Generalisability of results is compromised by small samples and lack of randomisation. Meagher et al. (1996) implemented eight nursing care strategies: at least 4-hourly observation; repeated orientation to surroundings; avoidance of excessive staff changes; use of a single room; uncluttered nursing environment; use of a night light; specific effort to minimise noise; and active encouragement of regular visiting by family and friends to help reorientate the person with delirium. The study found that nurses were least likely to care for a person with delirium in a single room, limit staff changes, reduce noise levels and involve relatives in care.

Lundstrom et al.'s (1999) intervention programme for patients with hip fracture consisted of education sessions, orthogeriatric liaison, improved multidisciplinary team working and a new rehabilitation care environment. There was a significant reduction in the incidence of delirium and fewer post-op complications, and a large proportion of patients returned to their own home as opposed to institutional care.

Inouye et al. (1999) initiated an interdisciplinary intervention consisting of a formalised programme using simple but measurable strategies with general medical patients. The intervention significantly reduced the incidence of delirium in the treated group where measures to promote sleep and mobility, correct vision, hearing and hydration were able to reduce the duration of delirious episodes but not the severity. Of note is that the higher the levels of adherence to the measures, the greater the reduction in the rates of delirium in a graded manner (Inouye et al., 2003).

Milisen et al. (2001) initiated a nurse-led interdisciplinary intervention programme to prevent delirium in hip-fracture patients. The intervention consisted of a nurse education programme, a nurse-resource scheme and scheduled administration of analgesia to every patient. Although there was no significant effect on the incidence of delirium, the duration and severity of delirium were reduced in the intervention group. There was no effect on functional status of patients or length of stay.

Experiential care evidence

Nurses can work effectively by anticipating that older people are at risk of developing delirium and developing a proactive culture of care. This entails an awareness that delirium can develop in an older person at any time if they have predisposing and precipitating risk factors. Delirium is an important focus for preventive and supportive care, particularly for nurses working in acute care and increasingly in other care settings. Lipowski (1990) describes the early warning signs of developing delirium that often occur during the night. The person wakes up just after a few hours of sleep, and seems restless, anxious and disorientated. The individual may have vivid dreams, hallucinations, or both, and may be uncertain if they have been dreaming, hallucinating or watching actual events. Prodromal signs such as these should raise the nurse's suspicion that the person may be developing delirium. In this situation, the person ideally needs the presence of a supportive individual who can respond with orientation to the ward and situation, and validation of the person's feelings in order to calm them if they seem frightened. The people in the scenarios remembered communication from nurses. A nurse's experience and clinical judgement will dictate what seems most appropriate.

The staff nurse of the orthopaedic ward in Case Study 14.6, for example, decides that validation of the person's feelings is most appropriate on this occasion. The nursing staff knew that the man's wife had died 3 years before and that it was the time of their anniversary. The nurse used this information in deciding how best to respond. Working to agreed protocols, nurses may be in a position to carry out clinical investigations in an effort to determine the cause of the delirium. The person in Case Study 14.7 had already been diagnosed with a chest infection, but the medical ward staff nurse's account of the care she provided and her reasons for giving it highlight the effectiveness of a calm and attentive approach. The success of this outcome was dependent on there being a nurse, carer or sitter with appropriate communication skills to sit with the confused person.

Case study 14.6

'He thought that I was somebody else and I didn't say, "No I'm the nurse, you're in hospital". And he kept calling me "Betty" and I said, "Yes darling". He said, "How's your mum" and I said, "She's absolutely fine, she's grand don't be worrying about her," and he was happy then. He said, "Oh thank God I was worrying about your mother, I thought something awful had happened to her." Now I think he was relating this maybe to his wife but he was showing it in different ways by being anxious about somebody else.'

Case study 14.7

'I very recently looked after an elderly woman who was transferred over from the local psychiatric hospital in an acute confusional state. She was very medically ill at the same time and she required one-to-one nursing. Because of her confusion she didn't understand that she needed to keep the oxygen on. She was pulling at her IV line, and she was pulling at her catheter. She didn't want any of it and she didn't understand why it was there. She didn't know she was in hospital and I think what really settled her was not that she was made to understand why she was here but that I got another nurse to sit with her. And it was just a case of holding her hand and we managed to keep the oxygen on, we managed to keep the fluids going and we managed to resolve all these things. She did have a chest infection so once we got on top of that, the confusion started to resolve. I think it was just basically spending time with her and making sure all these interventions went ahead, because the less oxygen she had the more hypoxic she was getting, the more confused she was getting so it was like a vicious circle. Just to screen off the rest of the environment and to get rid of the noise so that she wasn't seeing all the other people rushing about. She wasn't seeing other patients that were in the same room that were confused as well and just that she had the total attention of one person who was trying to reassure her'.

Although articles and delirium guidelines frequently advocate nursing patients with delirium in single rooms, these are not always available in

UK hospitals. Furthermore, nurse participants in an ongoing study stated a preference for nursing confused patients in multiple occupation rooms, as they were easier to monitor by the nurses themselves and other patients who would call for a nurse if a fellow patient seemed at risk of harm or if they felt threatened by the confused patient. By necessity, therefore, patients tend to be cared for in multiple-occupation rooms or wards, where their needs may be in conflict with those of fellow patients, as described by the nurse of the medical ward in Case Study 14.8.

Case study 14.8

'Very often it's at night that it's worse so that it keeps others off their sleep. They don't feel very well anyway and then when they have this sort of thing added. Other patients don't have a great deal of patience with it you know, which is understandable. Some patients with delirium get into quite a paranoid state, they're really anxious and think people are mistreating them and they're not in the right place and that sort of thing. They need extra reassurance but it doesn't always work. It's best to be honest with them and not treat them like children. Just try to explain that it's temporary that they are ill in hospital and try to explain the situation. It doesn't always work but sometimes it does though I think if they have really paranoid type behaviour then it doesn't always get through to them.'

The 'paranoid type behaviour' cited by staff nurse in Case Study 14.8 is likely to be triggered by powerful feelings and emotions which cannot be tempered by sensitive communication. In such situations, it is most appropriate to give sedation in order to calm and protect the person from harming themselves and others, relieve their distress and begin their medical treatment (British Geriatrics Society, 2005). There is a large amount of literature on the most appropriate type and dosage regimes of sedation for patients with delirium, although it is usually recommended that sedation is used as a last resort (British Geriatrics Society, 2005). There are many pressures, however, on nurses who work in multiple-occupation acute care settings, and where there is a lack of anticipatory and proactive care for confused patients, which is supported by senior managers, then nurses are likely to use sedation because they have no other option. Nurses feel duty-bound to act to protect the confused patient, other patients and sometimes themselves. In the absence of other supports such as sitters and the judicious use of electronic alarm systems, the use of sedation may be their only means of achieving this.

There is some evidence to suggest that on occasions, patients remember how they felt about behaviour over which they had no control during an episode of delirium (Schofield, 1997; McCurren and Cronin, 2003). Once the delirium has resolved, as in the case of the patient in Case Study 14.7, a person may feel very embarrassed and contrite about what they did. Nurses do not tend to routinely remind patients of their past behaviour in order to protect them from embarrassment. If a person raises the issue, it is appropriate, however, to provide some debriefing as to what was the likely cause of the delirium and to inform them that it is common for older people to experience this condition in the event of acute illness. It would have been appropriate to debrief the patient in Case Study 14.9 in this way (Case Study 14.9, staff nurse of the medical ward). Box 14.2 summarises the knowledge and skills essential to care for people with delirium.

Case study 14.9

'I've spoken to people who have had infections and some of them are really apologetic. Like when they find out they've thrown a jug of water over someone. It happened to one of the staff the other day, they had a jug of water thrown over them. It was just at the start of her shift and she knew it was completely out of character for this guy to do anything like that. They later found out he had a urinary tract infection and after a few days he was fine. But she never looked after him again. And then she got a card and a box of chocolates or something through the post with a huge apology saying "I'm so sorry, when I found out I was totally mortified". A lot of people just can't believe they were like that'.

Box 14.2   Summary of knowledge and skills essential to nurse people with delirium

- Knows defining features of delirium
- Knows the risk factors
- Anticipates that delirium may occur at any time and in any setting
- Uses a screening tool to diagnose delirium
- Listens carefully to the person with delirium
- Uses cues to interpret how the person with delirium might be feeling
- Communicates sensitively and clearly with the person who has delirium
- Advocates for the person with delirium
- Uses clinical judgement to decide on the most appropriate position in ward for the person with delirium and other patients
- Assertive in requesting resources for care, and e.g. sitters and electronic alarm systems
- Makes appropriate use of sedation
- Concurrently initiates clinical investigations to detect the underlying cause
- Works with colleagues to devise a permanent local protocol for care

Conclusion

Acutely ill, older people who are admitted to hospital are at risk of delirium. As the hospital population of older people is increasing steadily, it is likely that there will be a corresponding rise in the incidence and prevalence of delirium. This projected rise adds impetus for nurses to gain an understanding of the phenomenon and to practise proactive and supportive care that maintains the safety and dignity of older patients. There is currently a lack of knowledge of this commonly occurring phenomenon, especially as it affects the older person. This serves to minimise the significance of delirium to the individual concerned and compromises nurses' ability to advocate for the resources they need to provide quality care.

References

American Psychiatric Association (1994) *Diagnostic and Statistical Manual Of Mental Disorders*, 4th edn revised. Washington, DC, American Psychiatric Association.

British Geriatrics Society (2005) *Guidelines for the prevention, diagnosis and management of delirium in older people in hospital.* http://www.bgs.org.uk/Publications/Publication%20Downloads/Delirium-2006.DOC

Cole, M. (2004) Delirium in elderly patients. *American Journal of Geriatric Psychiatry* **12**, 7–21.

Faculty of Old Age Psychiatry, Royal College of Psychiatrists (2005) *Who Cares Wins.* London: Royal College of Psychiatrists.

Foreman, M. (1990) Cognitive and behavioural nature of acute confusional states. *Scholarly Inquiry for Nursing Practice: An International Journal* **5** (1), 3–16.

Inouye, S.K. (1999) Predisposing and precipitating factors for delirium in hospitalized older patients. *Dementia and Geriatric Cognitive Disorders* **10**, 393–400.

Inouye, S.K., Bogardus, S., Charpentier, P., Leo-Summers L., Acampora D., Holford T. and Cooney L. (1999) A multicomponent intervention to prevent delirium in hospitalized older patients. *New England Journal of Medicine* **340** (9), 669–676.

Inouye, S.K., Bogardus, S.T., Williams, C.S., Leo-Summers L. and Agostini, J.V. (2003) The role of adherence on the effectiveness of nonpharmacological interventions: Evidence from the delirium prevention trial. *Archives of Internal Medicine* **163**, 958–964.

Inouye, S.K. and Charpentier, P.A. (1996) Precipitating factors for delirium in hospitalized elderly persons: Predictive model and interrelationship with baseline vulnerability. *Journal of the American Geriatrics Society* **275**, 852.

Inouye, S.K., van Dyck, C.H., Alessi, C.A., Balkin, S., Siegal, A.P. and Horwitz, R.I. (1990) Clarifying confusion: the confusion assessment method, a new method for the detection of delirium. *Annals of Internal Medicine* **113**, 941–948.

Johnson, J. (1999) Identifying and recognizing delirium. *Dementia and Geriatric Cognitive Disorders* **10** (5), 353–358.

Lipowski, Z.J. (1990) *Delirium: Acute Confusional States.* New York: Oxford University Press.

Lundstrom, M., Edlund, A., Lundstrom, G. and Gustafson, Y. (1999) Reorganization of nursing and medical care to reduce the incidence of postoperative delirium and improve rehabiliation outcome in elderly patients treated for femoral neck fractures. *Scandinavian Journal of Caring Science* **13**, 193–200.

McCurren, C. and Cronin, S.N. (2003) Delirium: Elders tell their stories and guide nursing practice. *MEDSURG Nursing* **12** (5), 318–323.

Meagher, D.J., O'Hanlon, D., O'Mahoney, E. and Casey, P.R. (1996) The use of environmental strategies and psychotropic medication in the management of delirium. *British Journal of Psychiatry* **168**, 512–515.

Milisen, K., Foreman, M.D., Abraham, I.L., De Geest, S., Godderis, J., Vandermeulen, E., Fischler, B., Delooz, H.H., Spiessens, B. and Broos, P.L.O. (2001) A nurse led interdisciplinary intervention program for delirium in elderly hip-fracture patients. *Journal of the American Geriatrics Society* **49**, 523–532.

Milisen, K., Foreman, M.D., Wouters, B., Driesen, R., Godderis, J., Abraham, I.L. and Broos, P.L.O. (2002) Documentation of Delirium. *Journal of Gerontological Nursing* **28** (11), 23–29.

Neelon, V., Champagne, M.T., Carlson, J.R. and Funk, S.G. (1996) The NEECHAM Confusion Scale: construction, validation, and clinical testing. *Nursing Research* **45**, 324–330.

O'Keeffe, S. and Lavan, J. (1997) The prognostic significance of delirium in older hospital patients. *Journal of the American Geriatrics Society* **45**, 174–178.

O'Keeffe, S.T. (1999) Clinical subtypes of delirium in the elderly. *Dementia and Geriatric Cognitive Disorders* **10**, 380–385.

Sandberg, O., Gustafson, Y., Brannstrom, B. and Bucht, G. (1999) Clinical profile of delirium in older patients. *Journal of the American Geriatrics Society* **47**, 1300–1306.

Schofield, I. (1997) A small exploratory study of the reaction of older people to an episode of delirium. *Journal of Advanced Nursing* **25,** 942–952.

Schuurmans, M.J., Donders, R.T., Shortridge-Baggett, L.M. and Duursma, S.A. (2002) Delirium case finding: Pilot testing of a new screening scale for nurses. *Journal of the American Geriatrics Society* **50** (4, supplement S1–S204), S3.

Wolanin, M.O. and Phillips, L.R.F. (1981) *Confusion Prevention and Care*. St Louis, MO, Mosby.

Chapter 15
Enduring Mental Health Issues

Barry Aveyard

Introduction

The mental health care of older people with long-term enduring mental health conditions is an area of care that is often ignored and under-researched (Jolley et al., 2004). It is also recognised as a complex area in which to plan, commission and provide meaningful services for users. The report 'Everybody's Business' (Care Services Improvement Programme, 2005) highlighted the need to ensure there is recognition that older people with mental health needs can be supported by a variety of care agencies, and because of this, communication barriers can occur, resulting in people not receiving the support that they are entitled to. Arguably, this is a particular problem in the provision of services for older people with enduring mental health needs.

It is vitally important that care services acknowledge that older people can experience complex mental health needs. For example, it is not widely accepted that older people may have to cope with various forms of substance dependence. The case for clear comprehensive needs assessment is made by the Royal College of Psychiatrists (2002), who make it clear that without good communication between all involved in the provision of health services, some older people with enduring mental health conditions will become lost within the system.

This chapter will explore some of the major challenges involved in providing good-quality care in terms of both individualised care and provision of good-quality health and social care services. The chapter will focus upon the following major issues:

- schizophrenia;
- bipolar disorder;
- substance misuse.

The chapter will utilise case studies, which aim to illustrate some of the complex issues that arise in providing care for this client group, and how care needs can be best met. The case studies are intended to illustrate some of the challenges and dilemmas that arise when working with older people with enduring mental health conditions. They are intended to promote reflection on how these challenges might be met.

Schizophrenia

The stereotypical image of an older person with schizophrenia is perhaps someone who spent many years of their life in a large psychiatric institution and was discharged into some form of community care upon closure of the institution. While this is a real experience for many older people with schizophrenia, it is also important to acknowledge that some have lived successful lives in the community supported by family and friends. While for most people, schizophrenia manifests itself before the age of 45, the reality for some older people is that schizophrenia is a condition that does not develop itself until older age (Howard et al., 2000). Within the UK, it is suggested that schizophrenia might affect as many as 1% of the older population (Rodriguez-Ferra and Vassilas, 1998).

The National Institute for Health and Clinical Excellence (2002a) describes schizophrenia as a condition where people hear voices (hallucinations) and express ideas that other people do not agree with (delusions). They suggest that the condition is usually episodic in onset with people experiencing repeat acute exacerbations, although for some people, symptoms never fully go away, and they develop a chronic condition where even with treatment, they are never fully free of symptoms. It is this group of individuals who have a lifetime's experience of the condition who present the biggest challenges to care.

Treatment

The typical pharmacological treatment used is antipsychotic medication, and the basic action of this medication is unchanged since the 1950s, with the aim of treatment being to reduce or remove the experience of hallucinations and delusions. Some of the older medications still in use and recommended by the National Institute for Health and Clinical Excellence (2002b) have fairly significant side effects, including the possibility of drug-induced Parkinson's disease. There are newer 'atypical' antipsychotic medications that are less likely to cause such serious side effects, but they are more expensive and therefore not always prescribed as a first-choice intervention.

For many older people with schizophrenia and a long-term history of treatment with anti-psychotic medication, tardive dyskinesia is a significant issue. Tardive dyskinesia occurs late in the course of treatment (Jeste et al., 1999); it results in a dystonia of the brain and spinal cord, often resulting in involuntary and painful muscle contractions, which can cause abnormal body postures (Mind, 2004).

For many years, tardive dyskinesia was seen as an inevitable and unavoidable complication of the necessary drug interventions used in the management of schizophrenia. However, in reality, it is a devastating condition in its own right. For some, it has led to a loss of all ability to control voluntary movements, often resulting in the person not being able to keep their tongue in their mouth. While for some people the worst effects can be reduced with the use of medication such as Clonazepam, it has also been suggested that Vitamin E may help reduce the effects (Darton, 2004).

The reality is, however, that the condition is disabling in its own right, and more must be done through careful monitoring of medication use to prevent it developing in the first place.

Institutionalisation

The concept of the damage done to the ability to live independent lives caused by living in long-stay psychiatric hospitals was first described by Barton (1959). He developed the term 'Institutional Neurosis' as a way of describing the significant effects of living for many years in hospitals.

The reality for many people with schizophrenia was that they lived on wards in psychiatric hospitals, where virtually every life decision was made for them. They had no choice in when they got up in the morning, when they went to bed at night, what and when they ate and were often dressed in institutional clothing that was shared with others on the ward. For many, the long-term effects of institutionalisation had significantly more effect upon their quality of life than the effects of living with schizophrenia.

The closure of the large psychiatric hospitals throughout the 1990s brought about many positive changes in the care of people with long-term mental health conditions and did much to address issues of choice and autonomy. However, it is important to recognise that there are still people living in a variety of care settings who still experience the long-term effects of institutionalisation, and as such they can still have great difficulty when trying to make day-to-day decisions about living their lives.

Late-onset schizophrenia

Because schizophrenia is typically associated with being a condition which manifests itself in early adulthood, the notion that schizophrenia might develop in later life has not been fully recognised until recently. The classification has been suggested that late-onset schizophrenia is after the age of 40, and very late onset begins after the age of 60 (Howard et al., 2000).

It is generally accepted that late-onset schizophrenia will usually present with a significant paranoid element (McClure et al., 1999), and this can be misleading in terms of diagnosis of the condition. There can be assumptions made that anyone over the age of 60 who starts to behave in a way that is different for them is exhibiting signs of dementia. This point reinforces the importance of a full and accurate assessment when working with older people with suspected mental health conditions. It is perhaps too often the case that lack of thorough initial assessment leads to an inaccurate diagnosis and a significant delay in access to appropriate services and support. Clear guidance on the diagnosis of schizophrenia beyond the age of 60 is not easily accessible. The National Institute for Health and Clinical Excellence (2006) guidelines on schizophrenia are very comprehensive and give clear information for professionals on accurate diagnosis; however, they are aimed at people under the age of 60.

There is clear evidence to suggest a need to develop mental health services to ensure that people who develop schizophrenia in later life really do have access to the same services as those who develop the condition earlier in life (ReThink, 2004).

Case Study 15.1 highlights issues related to schizophrenia in later life and will assist in the understanding of some of the significant challenges associated with living with schizophrenia in later life.

Case study 15.1

Iris is 78 and lives in a nursing home with 24 other residents. Iris was admitted to a large 'psychiatric' hospital, in her late twenties, where she lived for many years until it was closed in the late 1980s. She lived for a few years with other residents with enduring mental health conditions in a 'hostel'.

During this time, she tended to neglect herself and became very withdrawn and uncommunicative. Through the support of a community mental health nurse, Iris was found a bed in the nursing home in the late 1990s. The home is run by a charity and cares exclusively for older people with enduring mental conditions. The qualified staff in the home all have a mental-health nursing qualification, the home has a good record of staff retention and staff are clearly motivated to provide the best care they can.

Iris has her own room with ensuite facilities but seems to prefer to sit in the communal day area of the home. She is very uncommunicative with both staff and other residents, she shows no interest in the television and newspapers and she will attend social events in the home but never participate. Iris often appears preoccupied and appears to respond to voices.

The issues within this case study are that Iris has no seeming interest in anything, other than eating, she is physically well cared for, but her mental well-being needs are not being met.

A case discussion in the home established the following issues:

- Little was known by staff of Iris's biography, yet no one had ever really talked to her about her past or looked at the extensive medical notes held within the home.
- Care staff were experienced but felt they had no real knowledge about schizophrenia as a condition or how to respond to someone hearing voices.
- Care staff admired the way qualified nurses responded to Iris but felt that they needed some education from the qualified staff so that they might be able to develop more skills.
- Staff were aware that there was a need to develop activities in the home beyond larger-scale events like bingo and beetle drives, but were unsure how to do this.

How were these issues addressed?

- Staff tried to develop a biography for Iris, and they realised that she was able to tell them a lot about her time in the psychiatric hospital and her life before admission.

- Iris had worked in the hospital gardens for many years and loved dogs.
- Qualified staff and researchers developed a teaching programme for care staff; sessions were based around individual residents and included discussion and teaching around the residents diagnosis as well as discussion of how care might be developed for each resident.

The results of these changes for Iris were:

- She started to go for walks with individual staff to a local park; while not communicating with staff in long conversations, she would often make comments about plants in the garden.
- A review of medication was undertaken with medical staff that supported the home, and as a result Iris appeared less troubled by voices.
- Staff started to feel more confident in working on an individual basis, having more knowledge about schizophrenia made them more aware of what Iris had experienced in her life and having a biography helped them to look at individualising her care.
- Ideas about activity changed, less focus was placed on group events, although these were available for those who wanted to take part, but more emphasis was placed on individual time for Iris.

This case study emphasises the importance of education and knowledge; staff cannot be expected to care for someone when they do not have an understanding of the impact of a condition like schizophrenia on an individual.

It also emphasises the value of sharing knowledge, the care staff had a great deal of information about Iris's day to day needs, and this was channelled into a more dynamic way of working with her through the case-study discussion.

Homelessness

It is thought that the numbers of older homeless people tend to be underestimated (Crane, 1998). For older people with mental health conditions, the link between mental health and homelessness may be more complex than is often recognised. Some older homeless people develop mental health conditions such as depression because they are homeless; for others, their mental health may be a contributing factor to their homelessness. Folsom et al. (2002) highlight that very few studies have examined the impact of schizophrenia on the lives of homeless people. However, they suggest that many people who are homeless and have schizophrenia will struggle to find appropriate high-quality mental health care. It is also suggested that there is a reluctance to admit older homeless people with schizophrenia into acute hospitals if they develop medical or surgical conditions.

There is perhaps a tendency for nurses and other health care workers to be naive in their work with older homeless people. It might be tempting to assume that all older homeless people fit into the category of 'vagrant' and potentially miss the fact that the person has unmet mental health needs.

Bipolar disorder

Bipolar disorder was historically referred to as manic depression, and while the term bipolar is now in general use, the term manic depression is still used by some people. Bipolar disorder is generally associated with mood swings, ranging from depressed to euphoric or manic behaviour. It is important to identify that the mood swings experienced by people with bipolar disorder are considerably more intense than the normal ups and downs most people experience (National Institute for Health and Clinical Excellence, 2003a).

The differing experiences of people with Bipolar disorder have been described by the support group Bipolar Aware (2001) in the following way:

Bipolar I:

- not the most common form of the illness;
- depression and intense episodes of mania;
- often long periods of stability;
- can have recurrent episodes of depression with one or two significant episodes of mania.

Bipolar II:

- recurrent depression and brief hypomanic episodes;
- elations are not as severe and are diagnosed as hypomania;
- hard to recognize because hypomania may seem normal if the person is very productive and does not cause problems for those around them.

Bipolar III:

- elations occur secondary to antidepressant medication;
- there is often a family history;
- some have manic episodes only (referred to as unipolar manic episodes).

Rapid Cycling:

- four or more episodes in one year;
- 'out of control', rollercoaster, yo-yo tendencies;
- in and out of hospital;
- difficult to achieve control with medication;
- 5–15% of all patients with bipolar disorders; 85% are female.

Like schizophrenia, bipolar disorder is a condition which usually develops in early adulthood but can in some cases develop in later life. Some older people with bipolar may have a long history of institutionalisation, whereas others will have a long history of support from family and friends, enabling them to live within the community. It has been suggested that bipolar among older people is an area lacking in research and knowledge (Depp and Jeste, 2004). It is an area that has not been seen as a priority; however, as life expectancy continues to grow, there will be more people living longer into old age with bipolar disorder, and there will be little evidence as to what their needs will be in terms of care and treatment.

Late-onset bipolar disorder

Late-onset bipolar disorder is often associated with organic brain disease (Kessing, 2006); however, there is a lack of detailed research which clearly contrasts the experiences of a person developing the condition in later life with a person developing the condition in young adulthood. It is generally accepted that a person developing the condition in later life will experience more manic episodes and be less prone to depression; however, the evidence for this may be more anecdotal than scientific.

Treatment

The basic components of pharmacological intervention involve three elements:

- antidepressants;
- antipsychotic medication;
- mood stabilisers.

Antidepressant medication is clearly indicated for someone in the depressive phase of the condition; there can be problems with the use of antidepressant medication because there is a risk that a person can be lifted from the depressive phase of the condition into the manic phase without a period of stability in between.

The use of antipsychotic medication is usual within the manic stage, as it has the potential to both reduce the delusional element of the condition and lower levels of euphoria. There is also the possibility of the medication lowering mood quickly into depression. However, the National Institute for Health and Clinical Excellence (2003a) recognises the role of the atypical antipsychotic drug, Olanzapine, as being useful in the treatment of bipolar disorder. It is regarded as having a role in both the control of mania and maintenance through its mood-stabilising properties.

Mood stabilisers were first used in the 1950s with the intention of lessening the problems highlighted above. Medications are defined as mood stabilisers if they have two distinct property functions:

- They provide relief from acute episodes of mania and depression, or prevent them from occurring.
- They do not worsen depression or mania, or lead to an increase in cycling (Hannant, 2001). Historically, anticonvulsant drugs such as Carbamazepine have been used as mood stabilisers or, more usually, the mood-stabilising drug, lithium. The National Institute for Health and Clinical Excellence (2003a) supported the use of the drug valproate semisodium; this is a development of

the anticonvulsant drug, sodium valproate, but is used as a mood stabiliser. The use of this drug is recommended because of the potential toxic side effects associated with lithium.

Electroconvulsive therapy

Electroconvulsive therapy (ECT) has a long history of use in mental health services. Dating back to the 1930s, it has traditionally been used in the treatment of severe depression, mania or schizophrenia. It essentially involves the passing of an electric current through the brain, which induces a seizure; this is done under anaesthetic while the patient is under the influence of a muscle relaxant (National Institute for Health and Clinical Excellence, 2003b). ECT has been used for some time and remains a controversial intervention, as there is little clear evidence as to how and why it works.

The National Institute for Health and Clinical Excellence (2003b) has guidance which recommends that ECT should only be used for severe enduring depression, catatonia or mania. It should be limited to gain fast short-term benefit when all other treatment options have failed or when the situation is considered to be life-threatening. Both Mind (2005) and the Social Care Institute for Excellence (2006) have suggested that ECT is used in excess for older people. This is despite the added risks to older people of ECT potentially causing cardiovascular problems.

It is clear that ECT is likely to remain a controversial treatment that divides opinion, although it clearly has its supporters among both health professionals and service users.

Substance misuse

Substance misuse is generally not perceived to be an issue among older people. Fingerhood (2000) highlighted that one of the issues in understanding the nature and extent of substance misuse among older people is that there is a limited amount of research available. This chapter will focus on substance abuse in terms of:

- alcohol;
- illicit drugs;
- prescription drugs.

Alcohol

Schofield and Tolson (2001) suggest that more attention must be paid to developing awareness of alcohol-related problems among older people. They argue that because of the physiological changes that occur with ageing, it is not sufficient to use the usually acceptable 'safe intake of alcohol limits' that are used with younger adults. Potentially, even small amounts of alcohol may have an impact upon an older person. They also highlight the importance of drug and alcohol interactions, as older people are more likely to use a wide range of prescribed medication; they are more likely to be susceptible to drug interactions. It is also important to recognise that for some older people, alcohol dependence is something that develops in later life; there are others for whom it is a problem that may have been part of their lives for many years. This group of people may have a different view of their drinking than someone for whom the problem is relatively new.

O'Connell et al. (2003) suggest that it can be quite hard to assess the alcohol consumption levels of older people. It may well be that older people are reluctant to discuss their alcohol consumption with health care workers. This of course may be the case for people of any age group; when asked by health professionals about their alcohol consumption, the usual answer for many people may be that they 'drink socially'. It is traditionally assumed that alcohol abuse is something that men are more likely to have problems with, but increasingly women are experiencing alcohol-dependence problems (Blow, 2000).

It is, perhaps easier for alcohol problems to be masked in older adults. An increase in falls, confusion or depression may well be attributed to other causes by health-care workers who are unsuspicious that alcohol dependence might be an issue. The result if often that older people with alcohol dependence receive treatment for several physical conditions without anyone becoming aware that alcohol is the cause of the problems (Beullens and Aertgeerts, 2004).

There may be a number of factors associated with alcohol misuse in older people (Dar, 2006); these tend to be grouped into three subheadings:

- emotional and social problems such as bereavement;
- medical problems, which may include issues such as cognitive impairment;
- practical problems including financial insecurity.

A clear and accurate assessment is not easy in this situation; many older people are unlikely to admit to a stranger on first meeting that they have an alcohol-dependence issue, if indeed they are aware themselves that they have alcohol dependence. One potential way forward is to highlight the need for mental health promotion for older people, and then health workers may become more aware that alcohol dependence may be an issue for some older people and that it is something that needs to be considered. Furthermore, depression screening may also play a valuable role, but all too frequently, assumptions are made that depression is normal among older people and therefore does not need thorough exploration. Greater awareness of the need to explore reasons behind depression may lead to more accurate detection of alcohol-dependence problems in older people.

Illicit drug abuse

Very little research-based knowledge is available about the extent and nature of illicit drug use among older people (Fingerhood, 2000). It is perhaps reasonable to assume that as a generation of regular illicit drug users age, there will be more older users of drugs like heroin or cannabis. It is suggested that as the 'baby boom' generation age there will be an increased use of illicit drugs amongst older people (Patterson et al., 1999). It is likely that health-care workers do not consider illicit drug abuse, as the assumptions of professionals may very well be that older people are unlikely to be illicit drug users.

Prescription drugs

Kaplan (2001) suggests that abuse of prescription drugs is an area of health care that needs further research, because of issues of polypharmacy and potential over prescribing of drugs among older people. Within the general population, abuse of prescription drugs has been described as a growing epidemic (Ayd, 1996). The true extent of prescription drug abuse among older people is difficult to gauge, and it is perhaps important to distinguish between substance misuse in terms of hoarding and storing drugs previously prescribed in case they are needed again or sharing drugs with other older people who may have similar symptoms (McGrath et al., 2005). This is a differing scenario to addiction to prescription drugs. One area of concern is addiction to benzodiazepines, often described as anxyiolitic drugs. They can help in the management of anxiety and sleep disorders and can be very useful if used under close supervision for short periods of time. However, the potential for addiction is high; some studies have suggested that it is common for older people to be prescribed these drugs for periods of 5 years or more (Widlitz and Marin, 2002).

While the need to monitor use and potential abuse of prescription medicines is clearly important, it is also necessary to be aware of the potential misuse of over-the-counter medication. Changes in legislation mean that there is an increasing range of medication now available over the counter in pharmacies or indeed from the shelf in shops and supermarkets.

There might be particular issues with:

- opioid-containing preparations (codeine);
- sleep aids;
- cough/cold medicines.

Pates et al. (2002) suggest that the role of local pharmacists in highlighting the problem is very important. However, this would not stop someone with a real addiction using several different pharmacies.

It is important that health-care staff are aware that, for some older people, drug abuse is a reality. Although it is a minority problem, it is a problem that could easily be missed through naivety or lack of thorough assessment by health-care workers.

Case Study 15.2 highlights the challenges of identifying the complex nature of working with older people with substance-misuse issues.

Case study 15.2

Nancy is 75 and lives in a small bungalow in a rural area on the edge of a large northern city. She was divorced from her husband many years ago and now lives alone. She is a member of the local church and worships every Sunday. She occasionally helps out at other church events but is not especially close to other church members.

Nancy enjoys a drink and has found supermarket own-brand gin very acceptable and well within her budget. She is aware that she is drinking a lot but never thinks of it as a problem. She has a lot of aches and pains and regularly buys Co-codamol tablets from the local pharmacy. She knows she takes a lot but is not sure how many she should take.

One Sunday in January, Nancy slips on her way out of church and falls in the church-yard. An ambulance is called, and Nancy is taken into hospital with a fractured neck of femur. Nancy has surgery to repair the injury.

In the days after the operation, Nancy is rather confused and difficult to nurse, often shouting at staff and other patients. She is overheard asking another visitor's relatives to buy her gin; this is seen as a little odd but attributed to her confusion.

A few days later, a visitor who knows Nancy a little from church speaks to a nurse. The visitor is awkward and unsure but feels she needs to tell someone. She says she maybe being nosey, but she is sure that Nancy is a drinker, there are rumours about her buying lots of gin in the local supermarket and she is sure she was drunk when she had her fall.

- How should the care team approach this information?
- Is it likely to be taken seriously or dismissed as gossip?
- How might Nancy be approached to discuss her drinking?
- Is it likely that her over-reliance on co-codamol might emerge in discussion?
- What agencies might need to be involved in this situation?

It is clear that this situation is more common and complex than health-care workers may be aware of. Many older adults who are alcohol-dependent may never receive any help because it is an issue that is under-researched and poorly understood.

However, in this situation, if the concern of a friend were dismissed or ignored, the situation might become worse, in terms of both alcohol withdrawal in hospital and a return to heavy drinking on discharge. It is imperative that, in this situation, some exploration of the situation takes place, even if the only way is to ask the individual about requesting others to buy them gin.

Conclusion

There has been a growing awareness of the mental health needs of older people in recent years, although the focus of this has been very much upon dementia. The work of organisations like the Alzheimer's Society has raised both public and professional awareness of the needs of people with dementia.

Awareness of other mental health conditions has some way to go. The reasons for this may be linked to the fact that within society in general, the conditions discussed in this chapter still carry with them a significant degree of social stigma. It may also be that their position within policy initiatives like National Service Frameworks is unclear and lacking in priority. For all the conditions described, the amount of research-based knowledge is clearly lacking, and as a result it is difficult to implement good-quality evidence-based care.

It is clear that health-care workers need to raise their own levels of knowledge and understanding, as these conditions have a significant impact upon the lives of older people, and this impact can easily be underestimated if professionals do not have the knowledge and skills to provide the complex support that is often needed.

References

Ayd, F.J. (1996) Prescription drug abuse and dependence: How prescription drug abuse contributes to the drug abuse epidemic. *The Journal of Nervous and Mental Disease* **184** (5), 329.

Barton, R. (1959) *Institutional Neurosis*. Bristol, UK, Wright.

Beullens, J. and Aertgeerts, B. (2004) Screening for alcohol abuse and dependence in older people using DSM criteria: a review. *Aging and Mental Health* **8** (1), 76–82.

Bipolar Aware (2001) *What is bipolar disorder?* www.bipolaraware.co.uk/whatisithtml

Blow, F.C. (2000) Treatment of older women with alcohol problems: Meeting the challenges for a special population. *Alcoholism Clinical and Experimental Research* **24** (8), 1257–1266.

Care Services Improvement Programme (2005) *Older people's mental health is Everybody's Business*. Leeds, UK, Care Services Improvement Programme.

Crane, M. (1998) The associations between mental illness and homelessness among older people: an exploratory study. *Aging and Mental Health* **2** (3), 171–180.

Dar, K. (2006) Alcohol use disorders in elderly people: fact or fiction. *Advances in Psychiatric Treatment* **12**, 173–181.

Darton, K. (2004) *Tardive Dyskinesia*. London, Mind.

Depp, C.A. and Jeste, V. (2004) Bipolar disorder in older adults: a critical review. *Bipolar Disorders* **6**, 343–367.

Fingerhood, M. (2000) Substance abuse in older people. *Journal of the American Geriatrics Society* **48**, 995–2000.

Folsom, D.P., McCahill, M., Bartels, S.J., Lindamer, L.A., Ganiats, T.G. and Jeste, D.V. (2002) Medical co morbidity and receipt of medical care by older homeless people with schizophrenia or depression. *Psychiatric Services* **53** (11), 1456–1460.

Hannant, M. (2001) *Information about medication*. http://www.bipolaraware.co.uk/medications.html

Howard, R., Rabins, P.V., Seeman, M.V. and Jeste, D.V. (2000) Late-onset schizophrenia and very-late-onset schizophrenia-like psychosis: An international consensus. *American Journal of Psychiatry* **157** (2), 172–176.

Jeste, D.V., Larco, J.P., Palmer, B., Rockwell, E., Harris, J. and Caligiuri, M.P. (1999) Incidence of tardive dyskinesia in early stages of low dose treatment with typical neuroleptics in older patients. *American Journal of Psychiatry* **156** (2), 309–326.

Jolley, D., Kosky, N. and Holloway, F. (2004) Older people with long-standing mental illness: the graduates. *Advances in psychiatric treatment* **10**, 27–36.

Kaplan, A. (2001) Trying to solve the prescription drugs abuse equation. *Psychiatric Times* **19** (2), 60–63.

Kessing, L.V. (2006) Diagnostic subtypes of bipolar disorder in older versus younger adults. *Bipolar Disorders* **8**, 56–64.

McClure, F.S., Gladsjo, J.A. and Jeste, D.V. (1999) Late-onset psychosis: Clinical, research, and ethical considerations. *American Journal of Psychiatry* **156** (6), 935–940.

McGrath, A., Crome, P. and Crome, I.P. (2005) Substance misuse in the older population. *Post Graduate Medicine* **81**, 228–231.

Mind (2004) *Making Sense of Antipsychotics (Major Tranquillisers)*. London, Mind.

Mind (2005) *Access All Ages*. London, Mind.

National Institute for Health and Clinical Excellence (2002a) *Schizophrenia: Information for the Public*. London, National Institute for Health and Clinical Excellence.

National Institute for Health and Clinical Excellence (2002b) *Guidance on the Use of Newer Atypical Antipsychotic Drugs for the Treatment of Schizophrenia*. London, National Institute for Health and Clinical Excellence.

National Institute for Health and Clinical Excellence (2003a) *Bipolar Disorder: New Drugs Guidance*. London, National Institute for Health and Clinical Excellence.

National Institute for Health and Clinical Excellence (2003b) *Electro Convulsive Therapy: Information for the Public*. London, National Institute for Health and Clinical Excellence.

National Institute for Health and Clinical Excellence and National Collaborating Centre for Mental Health (2006) *Schizophrenia Full Guidance*. London, Gaskell and the British Psychological Society.

O'Connell, H., Chin, A., Cunningham, C. and Lawlar, B. (2003) Alcohol disorders in elderly people redefining an old problem in old age. *British Medical Journal* **327**, 664–667.

Pates, R., McBride, A., Li, S., Ramadan, R. (2002) Misuse of over-the-counter medicines' survey of community pharmacies in a South Wales health authority. *The Pharmaceutical Journal* **268**, 179–182.

Patterson, T.L., Larco, J.P., Jeste, D.V. (1999) Abuse and misuse of medications in the elderly. *Psychiatric Times* **16** (4), 54–55.

ReThink (2004) *Lost and Found: Voices from the Forgotten Generation*. Kingston on Thames, UK, ReThink.

Rodriguez-Ferra, S. and Vassilas, C.A. (1998) Older people with schizophrenia: providing services for a neglected group. *British Medical Journal* **317**, 293–294.

Royal College of Psychiatrists (2002) *Council Report: Caring for People who Enter Old Age with Enduring or Relapsing Mental Illness ('Graduates')* London, Royal College of Psychiatrists.

Schofield, I. and Tolson, D. (2001) The nurse's role in assessing alcohol use by older people. *British Journal of Nursing* **10** (19), 1260–1268.

Social Care Institute for Excellence (2006) *Practice Guide: Assessing the Mental Health Needs of Older People*. http://www.scie.org.uk/publications/practiceguides/bpg2/index.asp

Widlitz, M. and Marin, D.B. (2002) Substance abuse in older adults. *Geriatrics* **57** (12), 29–34.

Chapter 16
Depression in Later Life

Jill Manthorpe and Steve Iliffe

Introduction

'*When depression hits me the last thing I want to do is to see the doctor, because it seems hard to define anything as 'wrong''* (Fanthorpe, 1996, p. 52). Depression is the commonest mental health condition in later life, and every nurse working with older people in the community, care homes or hospital services will encounter it on a weekly, if not daily, basis. At least one in ten people aged 65 or more has significant symptoms of depression like sadness, loss of energy, difficulties sleeping (Sharma and Copeland, 1989), persistent tiredness, headaches or widespread muscular aches and pains or poor concentration and memory. Most make regular contact with the health service, seeing their GP and practice nurse both for their depression symptoms and for long-term management. A systematic review of studies of older people living in the community aged 55 years and over suggests that minor depression affects about 13.5%, but depression in its most severe forms is less likely, about 1.8% (Beekman et al., 1999).

The 'physical' symptoms of depression may not be recognised for what they are (Watts et al., 2002). People with illness or disabilities that limit their capability to deal with the tasks of everyday life are more likely to be depressed than those who are more independent. High rates of depression are found among users of home care services (Patmore, 2002), and people who have just moved into a care home are particularly vulnerable to depression (Bagley et al., 2000). Poverty and depression go together (Beekman et al. 1999), and poorer and less-educated older people are less likely to seek help or treatment (Mills and Edwards 2002). Overall, depression is commoner in older women than in older men (Beekman et al., 1999). Lastly, there is evidence that mistreatment and neglect, including self-neglect, are associated with depression (Dyer et al., 2000).

Recent evidence from the first wave of the English Longitudinal Study of Ageing (ELSA) (Office of the Deputy Prime Minister, 2006), a large-scale survey of people aged 50 and over, found that depression has the widest influence over seven key dimensions of social exclusion. In each of the dimensions of social exclusion, except possession of material goods, being depressed was strongly related to the likelihood of having a poor quality of life. This makes it more important than age by itself, more important than poor health or living alone, being from an ethnic minority or having a low income. Addressing depression and mental health conditions is clearly going to be key in tackling the multiple exclusions that severely affect about 7% of people aged over 50.

What is depression?

'Energy is gradually returning and with it increased focus and perhaps a self-confidence that it is repairing itself. My depression could be worse, my demon more angry. Yet I remain fragile and need my refuge. There is nevertheless a desire to move out of my existing victim status . . . Doom does not overwhelm me, but remains my back-drop every hour of the day.' (Eastman, 2005; pp. 7–8)

All nurses working with older people need to be aware of the risk of depression, and while not everyone will specialise in mental heath, everyone should recognise the signs that might suggest that a specialist mental health assessment should be undertaken. Similarly, all nurses should be able to think about ways in which they can contribute to prevention of depression among older people, and also among carers and their colleagues. How can we distinguish between depression and sadness in a practical way? The following must be present for a diagnosis of depression to apply:

- *Duration*: Symptoms of depression (see Box 16.1) are present for at least 2 weeks. This time limit is arbitrary, but it is a time frame for the kinds of sadness that are triggered by ordinary life events in later life, like bereavement, illness and failure.
- *Lack of fluctuation*: Symptoms of depression occur most of the time on most days, a person is not likely to be distracted, and 'good days' (or even periods of the day) are few.
- *Intensity*: The severity of depression symptoms must be of a degree that is definitely not normal for that individual, so that they say 'I have never felt this bad before', or describe greater tiredness than usual in a busy life, frequent insomnia or greater difficulties getting to sleep and staying asleep than in the past, and so on. Carers or family members are key informants here, but so too are care workers and health professionals who know a person well.

This helps to separate understandable sadness from depression, but it does not indicate which symptoms are the key signs of depression, and which are possible signs but not diagnostic. The key symptoms of depression are as shown in Box 16.1.

Other symptoms that suggest depression include:

- suicidal thoughts or behaviour, such as thinking that life is hopeless, and the family would be better off without them or behaving in a way that seems to illustrate such thought, for example, cutting social ties or hoarding medicines or making an attempt to harm themselves;
- loss of confidence or self-esteem;
- feeling of helplessness;

Box 16.1   Key symptoms of depression (Alexopoulos et al., 2001)

> An individual has depression if any of the following three criteria apply:
> - They have a depressed mood sustained for at least 2 weeks (on most days, most of the time); AND/OR
> - They have lost interest or pleasure in usual activities ; AND/OR
> - They report decreased energy, increased fatigue (in patients who are physically ill this may mean feelings of fatigue, even when not attempting exertion) or diminished activity.

- inappropriate or excessive feelings of guilt;
- feelings of hopelessness or worthlessness;
- avoiding social interactions or going out;
- poor concentration and/or difficulty with memory;
- physical slowing or agitation (restlessness or fidgeting);
- sleep disturbance (particularly waking in the early hours and not being able to return to sleep);
- reduced appetite with corresponding weight loss.

While this seems clear when written down, it is much more difficult when encountering an old person in distress in Accident and Emergency, someone recovering from major surgery or an old person being treated at home for a leg ulcer. There are two traps for the nurse who comes to the conclusion that the older person they are working with is depressed. The first trap is that medical treatments work for some older people with depression, but not all, and even when they relieve the symptoms, the risk of relapse is high. A rule of threes has been suggested: that a third of older people with depression get better, a third remain the same and a third get worse (suggested initially by Millard, 1983 and confirmed by Chew-Graham et al., 2004). Expectations of 'cure' can be raised in discussing with someone why they should seek help for their depression, only to be disappointed when treatments have little or no effect. The second trap is that doctors and nurses may not always share the same clinical perspective on depression, with its rules about patterns of symptoms. A lot of a nurse's effort and negotiating skills can go into persuading a reluctant older person to describe their feelings and symptoms to a doctor, only to find that the doctor does not recognise the problem as depression at all. It is important to understand how these problems arise, and what can be done about them, by thinking about the problem of recognition further.

Depression is often missed (Audit Commission, 2000) and sometimes hidden. Studies of older people living at home show that it is under-diagnosed and under-treated (Garrard et al., 1998). Care home staff often fail to consider depression among residents, even if they are a qualified nurse (Bagley et al., 2000). Depressed people may think of admitting to depression as a weakness and so avoid stigma, and may divert attention from the mental health need to physical explanations. Nurses may find themselves responding to the headache, sleeplessness, back pain or other symptoms, rather than thinking about the underlying disturbances of thinking and emotion that may bind the

Box 16.2   Common tests for depression

Local services will use standard tests. They are likely to be any of the following:
● The 15-item Geriatric Depression Score (GDS15) or its four item version (GDS4);
● The Hospital Anxiety & Depression scale (HAD);
● The PHQ-9 Depression Scale (now being introduced into general practice).

symptoms together. This may apply to carers, whose risk of depression is high, particularly if their sleep is broken (Highet et al., n.d.), if they are supporting someone with dementia (Moriarty and Webb, 2000), if they want to give up caring (Levin et al 1994) or if their own health is poor (Moriarty and Webb, 2000). A carer's distress with lack of support may be real, but it is important to note the potential for a carer to be depressed and for this to affect perceptions of the adequacy of support.

Many care home residents have symptoms of depression. From the USA, we have evidence that it is possible to improve the accuracy of assessment and diagnosis of high-risk groups, such as people who move into nursing homes (Boyle et al., 2004) and that treatment is worth while. This seems to be shifting the longstanding pattern of under-recognition of depression, but such initiatives need to be followed through to make sure that treatment is working and that sustained attention makes sure that reassessment and monitoring occur. Box 16.2 highlights the common tests used for depression.

These tests are not diagnostic; they simply increase the probability that an individual who scores in the 'depression' ranges of each test is more likely to have these conditions. None of them can replace clinical judgment (Manthorpe and Iliffe, 2005a).

Case Study 16.1 illustrates how a diagnosis of depression could be 'missed' because his symptoms are misattributed to other causes, or the older person wants to avoid the diagnosis itself. It highlights the importance of making links between presenting behaviour, emotional state, physical assessment and patterns of social interaction (see Neal et al., 2001).

Case study 16.1

Mr A is 69, lives alone in a rented flat and remains well despite his 15-year history of hypertension and his more recent onset of angina. He takes medication for blood pressure control (Amlodipine, 10 mg daily), reduction of angina (ISMN, 20 mg daily) and to reduce his cholesterol (Simvastatin, 20 mg daily). He attends the practice nurse's follow-up clinic every 4 months for blood-pressure checks, review of symptoms and, when necessary, blood tests. During these consultations he often talks about his many aches and pains, and the nurse always suggests that he sees one of the doctors to investigate this further, but he never makes an appointment, saying when asked that he does not think the doctors can do anything for him. Mr A was a building worker and had moved to the UK in his twenties, to seek work. He has never married and has slowly lost contact with his family. He has struggled successfully to give up tobacco and no longer likes to socialise in the pub at weekends.

What should the practice nurse do? It would be tempting, with a large case-load and busy clinics, to do nothing more, on the grounds that advice has been given, and Mr A's autonomy has to be respected – he need not see a doctor about his symptoms if he does not want to. We have sympathy with this response, but there are better alternatives. One would be to alert Mr A's usual GP, so that the symptoms can be raised when Mr A next attends for something else – perhaps for his annual medication review. Another would be for the nurse to ask Mr A some questions about energy, fatigue, sleep patterns and enjoyment, using the diagnostic criteria described above. If he has these problems and is willing to talk about them, it may be possible for the nurse to raise the possibility that he is becoming depressed with him. Naming the problem can sometimes bring a sense of relief, but we have to be aware of the stigma associated with depression and not talk about a possible diagnosis too swiftly. This is a sensitive aspect of the practice nurse's work, but her background knowledge of the individual and the continuity of their relationships can be powerful assets. Assessed needs can only be met effectively if services are acceptable to the individual: this means that they must fit language, cultural, religious and spiritual expectations of the individual (Bracken et al., 1998). Mr A, for example, might think that depression is a sign of moral weakness or self-indulgence, and focus on physical symptoms and anyone trying to work with him will need to accept that his views differ from their own perception.

Depression and disability commonly go together, but we should be aware of stereotypes that see older people with disabilities as inevitably depressed. The shortage of long-term studies of depression in the community (Katona, 1989) and the different ways of selecting samples and measuring and identifying depression mean we have a wealth of studies but have to make sense of them in our own working contexts. What we do know is that the association between poor health and depression appears to be greater for those aged 75 and over, and for men, than for younger old people (aged 65–74 years) as a whole, or for women. Poor health, loss of mobility and depression are linked with loneliness and social isolation (Cattan, 2002), so nurses working with older men who are living alone should be conscious of their risk of depression. But how people feel about their lives and themselves also matters; subjective measures of ill-health like pain, or self-rating of overall healthiness and well-being, are more strongly related to depression than are more objective measures of illness or disability like the number of diseases or the degree of disability (Beekman et al., 1995). Opportunities for thinking about older people's mental health are likely to be greater, now we have more medication reviews and registers of people in primary care who have long-term conditions that need systematic follow-up and active medical management. Expert patient groups may allow people with disabilities to increase their control over their symptoms and lives, which may reduce the risk of depression. Knowledge of what groups do and how to contact them should be part of the nurse's role. Opportunities for brief discussions about morale, mood and coping may be taken at checks for diabetes, heart disease, chronic obstructive pulmonary disease and hypertension, but also when people come for influenza immunisations or other preventive care.

Depression and dementia

Memory loss is common in depression, and so depression can be easily mistaken for dementia. Moreover, half of people with dementia have depressive symptoms (Gottfries, 2001). The depression may last for many months (Ballard et al., 1996) and may occur at any stage of the dementia process. The impact of depression on top of cognitive impairment matters because it can cause much distress in early dementia and can trigger behavioural disturbances later. The result can be a vicious cycle of isolation and distress. One way for a nurse to assess this is to compare previous and current social support. This may be possible to do by using the information collected by the primary care team or social services, and thinking about it methodically, such as by use of a map of social support (like an ecogram). More likely, talking to one or more key informants may help provide clues about a possible change in social support, if the older person is not able to comment on this. Does the home care worker have anything to say about a reduction in social contacts? Has she seen visitors sent 'on their way'? How does the support plan or care plan reflect this? All these pointers will enable the care team to consider change and not to take previous support for granted.

Depression coexists with dementia so frequently that any person with dementia should be considered as possibly having a dual diagnosis at some stage (Manthorpe and Iliffe, 2006). As services stand at the moment, a diagnosis of dementia may take precedence over other mental health needs or cause them to be overlooked. This helps explain why depression is less commonly talked about than dementia and less commonly addressed in any care or treatment setting. It is worth trying antidepressant medication for a person with dementia who has depression.

Many professionals and family members are worried that telling a person that they have dementia will lead them to be depressed (Marzanski, 2000). Ways in which the risk of a depressive response to the diagnosis can be minimised are by providing support, and also by being aware that depression may have been an early feature of dementia, and so it is not the diagnosis disclosure itself that may 'cause' depression.

Features that may be common to dementia and depression (Cheston and Bender, 1999) include being withdrawn, forgetfulness, tearfulness and being in low spirits. Table 16.1 sums up some of the key differences (Alzheimer's Society, 2001). Communication as a way to gather information is important, assessment tools can be helpful and ways of assessing risk may be part of the long-term thinking and planning processes. In practice, one of the complications is the mistaking of dementia for depression and vice versa, and not thinking that the two might coexist. Case Study 16.2 illustrates this.

Table 16.1 Key differences between depression and dementia

	Dementia	Depression
Onset	Usually insidious	Gradual
Duration	Months/years	Weeks/months
Course	Progressive	Worse in mornings, improves during day
Alertness	Usually normal	Normal
Orientation	Usually impaired for time/place	Usually normal
Memory	Impaired recent, remote memory sometimes impaired	Recent may be impaired, remote is intact
Thoughts	Slowed, with reduced interests	Usually slowed, preoccupied with sad thoughts
Perception	Often normal	Congruent with mood
Emotions	Shallow, apathetic, labile, irritable	Flat, unresponsive, sad, fearful
Sleep	Often disturbed	Early-morning wakening

Case study 16.2

Mr B pottered about at home after his retirement, spending hours tending his garden as well as competing with his wife in the kitchen. Although he had never been a very sociable man and at times had seemed moody and morose, he seemed to enjoy the quietness of his life. Sometime shortly after his 74th birthday, his wife noticed that his passion for cooking had changed, and as the subsequent months passed, he did less and less, largely giving up gardening as well as cooking. He became irritable with his neighbours, shouting at them over the garden fence at the smallest provocation, and they began to complain to his wife. It was this change in his behaviour that prompted Mrs W to ask the specialist nurse for older people who worked in the local health centre what was happening to her husband, and in particular if he was getting depressed.

The specialist nurse for older people talked to Mrs B about her concerns when she saw them both and asked some questions about why she thought depression might be the problem. She wanted to know if Mr B was forgetting things, why he had stopped cooking, whether it was forgetting or not understanding recipes and whether he had been like this in the past when his mood was low. She listened to what Mr B had to say, how he was behaving and what he looked like, to make an accurate record of him as possible. Did he initiate conversation? How was he sleeping? Was he feeling any aches or pain? How was he eating? Had he lost any weight recently? What had he been doing in his day? 'How was he feeling in himself?' Did he think there were any problems with his levels of energy? Mr B confessed he was feeling that his confidence was ebbing away, that life was very sad at times and that he did not find that things gave him much pleasure any more. His eyes watered, and he blew his nose, saying it was hay fever.

In this assessment, the nurse was trying to find out if this was a new pattern or a repetition of an old pattern, if new, she would be thinking it might possibly indicate dementia. On leaving Mr B, she said she would like to talk to his GP about this visit, and Mr B said she could do as she wished. She took her conclusions back to the GP, since details of his past health concerns would help the primary care team gain a more complete picture, such as what was his 'premorbid' personality like, and had he coped with adverse events well before?

The nurse who visited Mr and Mrs B made the point of saying that Mrs B could contact her if she felt she needed to talk. Carer stress does seem to be reduced by knowledge that support is available, even if it is never taken up.

Depression and risk

'I have been in this home for five years. I had depression for two years, I was ill and I kept taking pills and they were making me worse . . . I ended up taking an overdose and ended up in hospital' (Janet Nelson, in Owens and National Care Homes Research and Development Forum, 2006).

Is it possible to think about depression as an iceberg, with most minor depression among older people undetected, but larger in scale? When depression is visible, it may be because it causes a crisis in the person's life or system of support, and in very serious instances the older person may consider that life is no longer worth living and take active steps to end their own life. In the UK, one in every eight people who commit suicide is aged 65 years and over, and men aged over 75 years have the highest rate of suicide of any age groups. These are not just concerns for the UK, for the high and rising rates of suicide occur globally among older people. Depression in later life is associated with disproportionately high rates of suicide and high death rates from all other medical causes (Montano, 1999; O'Connell et al., 2004).

About one in eight of all suicides in the UK are by older people, and most, 80%, commit suicide on apparently their first attempt (de Leo et al., 2001). Nevertheless, overall, suicide in later life is an uncommon event. The National Suicide Prevention Strategy report (Department of Health, 2002) welcomes the fall in numbers. Local implementation groups have been tasked with implementation of such strategies and are a good source of advice about the networks of local services for those who have made attempts and those who have been affected by a death by suicide.

Case Study 16.3 highlights the importance of being aware of the issues related to suicide when caring for older people.

Case study 16.3

Miss C has been admitted to hospital following a fall. She says she is in pain, especially at night, and she was very confused on admission. She is not happy with her care on the ward, saying that she is disturbed by the other patients, that the food is difficult to eat and cold and that the rehabilitation is bullying. She refuses to get up some times, and some of the nursing staff find it difficult to understand her but think this is connected to her pain.

K has been asked to pay particular attention to Miss C. She starts by spending some time with Miss C, asking her if she would like her bedside cupboard tidied up and if she can help her with personal care. She pulls the bedside curtains round to give greater privacy. Miss C outlines her problems with the ward and the other patients, who she finds disturb her, and the lack of traditional nursing care that she had expected. She is unforthcoming about herself to start with and more concerned with the harsh treatment she feels she is receiving.

Case study 16.3   (Continued)

K persists gently and does find out more about Miss C, an independent woman who has never faced such a hard knock to her confidence and who is greatly worried that she will be 'put in a home'. She says that life is hopeless, that she will never get better and that it is dreadful that she is taking up a bed when someone else should have it who is in greater need. She says that she just feels like ending it all.

K discusses this with the staff nurse. K says she knows that disability and depression are linked but says that it seems a chicken-and-egg situation to her. She thinks that Miss C's depression may be impairing her functioning, but she can see that Miss C's disability may be like bereavement at the loss of her former active self. Miss C does appear to have coped well until her fall but now seems overwhelmed. She is worried by Miss C's talk of guilt and her hopelessness.

The staff nurse does take this seriously, because Miss C has expressed guilt and because she has raised the possibility that she might take her own life. She makes sure that K records what she remembers of the conversation and makes a referral to the mental health liaison nurse. She suggests that K reflects on this case, and offers her time to talk about her feelings of responsibility and inability to make things better immediately for Miss C. The nursing care plan is revised to ask other staff to be patient with Miss C and to record sleep patterns and feelings. A dietary sheet is started to record food-and-drink intake. An early referral is made to the hospital social work team, asking them to start a community care assessment and advising them that Miss C is worried about being forced into a care home.

The associated risk factors for suicide are complex and overlapping, and sometimes not amenable to change. Focusing on one risk factor is unlikely to be helpful, and interventions are limited in efficacy and availability. There is no accurate way to identify people who are going to take their own lives, and all professionals live with this uncertainty. Any potential risk-assessment instrument would be too crude and would give far too many 'false positives' – people who will not kill themselves despite having the risk factor – to be practical or ethical. A further problem with risk factors is that they are open to bias or the benefit of hindsight. For example, a relative may assume that the older person who have killed themselves were depressed and describe their behaviour in the period before death in these terms because this seems a sensible explanation, but it may not be correct. With this caution, we should bear risk factors in mind because they do provide some useful clues (see Manthorpe and Iliffe, 2005b).

Risk factors contribute to an overall picture of an individual. Depression is common among people who take their own lives in old age (Harwood et al., 2001; Beautrais, 2002). Another set of risk factors surrounds physical ill health or disability (Harwood et al. 2000) or people's perceptions of this. Pain, lack of sleep (Turvey et al., 2002) and the onset of sight problems (Waern et al., 2002) are also proposed as possible risk factors.

For older people, focusing on prescribing may be the most important prevention strategy, since drug over-dose is the most common single method of suicide among older people. Harwood et al. (2000) suggest that doctors should reduce the prescription of combination analgesics. Hoarding medication is common, and not a suicide risk in itself, but a supply of drugs may be a means to suicide, so regular efforts to collect and dispose of unused medication make sense.

Treatment of depression

'Older people who have mental health problems have access to integrated mental health services, provided by the NHS and councils to ensure effective diagnosis, treatment and support for them and their carers' (Section 7 of the National Service for Older People; Department of Health, 2001).

There are three main ways to treat depression: social support, psychological therapies of various sorts and antidepressant medication. They are not mutually exclusive, and there is some evidence that a combination can work better than either alone (Baldwin et al., 2003). Some older people find it difficult to express their distress in psychological language, while others see antidepressant medication as dangerous, potentially addictive and a false solution for their problems. Social support and activities may not be what some depressed older people want, and they will not enjoy them. The kinds of therapies used need to be negotiated with each person, and this means listening to what the older person wants, thinks, and believes.

Offering support to depressed older people is associated with higher rates of recovery (in the sense of freedom from symptoms) (Baldwin et al., 2003). The community nurse visiting an older person for 20 minutes twice a week to attend to a leg ulcer may be an antidepressant without knowing it, simply by showing an interest in the older person's experience, life story, and well-being, relieving anxieties about coping or lifting loneliness. These kinds of personal relationships may restore a sense of worth that has been eroded. Even brief encounters with an empathic and experienced person may help the depressed individual to assimilate losses (developing compensatory mechanisms like new friendships) or to accommodate to them by changing expectations and standards. Active interventions coordinated and implemented at primary-care level by nurses seem to be effective in reducing depression (Blanchard et al., 2004).

Professional intervention may be a necessary response to worsening depression in an older person, but determining the type of treatment can be difficult. Social support seems to work by altering the thinking and feeling of older people in positive, antidepressant ways, but it is not usually consciously psychological: it is simply what people do in productive and reciprocal human relationships (see Battison, 2004 for a good guide). Psychotherapy is different because it is deliberate, framed in terms of psychological theories, frequently conducted on a one-to-one basis outside 'normal' relationships and often intense. Psychological treatments such as those recommended by the National Service Framework for Older People (Department of Health, 2001) (Cognitive Behaviour Therapy, Inter-Personal Therapy and brief focal analytic psychotherapy) are effective treatments but are underused (Burns et al., 2001). In general, cognitive therapy, the expansion of which is being advocated (Layard, 2004), suggests that similar treatments apply, regardless of age, but that certain factors need to be considered. These include the possibility that treatment needs to be at a slower pace (Wilkinson, 1997), that sessions may need to have greater structure, and that ideas should be less abstract. Other factors, such as taking account of hearing loss and the need for settings to be accessible and comfortable for those with disabilities such as joint pain also need considering. Age should not be a barrier to referring an older person for psychological therapies, but they are widely underused (Lebowitz et al., 1997; Burns et al., 2001). Local knowledge of such services' accessibility and thresholds is important for nurses.

Medical treatments

Prescribing antidepressants is largely a medical task, and even a nurse with prescribing powers will likely cross-check with the doctor, but understanding the ways in which they can help and should be used is everyone's responsibility starting with the person concerned. A treatment approach to optimise use of medication in the right doses requires:

- The choice of medication with low risks of adverse effects.
- A dialogue that elicits specific concerns about medication. The fear that antidepressants will not alter the underlying disease process is in one sense realistic, but most people in pain would not avoid taking pain relief because it does not heal the cause of the pain, so a discussion that rebadges depression as a symptom worth relieving is sensible. On the other hand, anxiety about becoming dependent on antidepressants is very reasonable, given the initial assurances that antidepressants are not habit-forming and the current concerns that they can be difficult to stop.

It is important to know why some treatments are chosen, as nurses may need to monitor their use, look out for side effects and assess response. For example, antidepressants in the Selective Serotonin Re-uptake Inhibitor (SSRI) family can, in some people, increase agitation and sleeplessness or cause dizziness, so their use needs careful monitoring, particularly at the start of treatment. Nurses should also talk to people about their feelings and fears about medication. The choice and use of antidepressant medication should be based on the principles shown in Box 16.3.

Treatment depends on personal history, other medical problems, and the person's preferences; but the nature and depth of the depression also matter. An approach to deciding on treatment options for the different types of depressive disorder developed by the Royal College of Psychiatrists Faculty of Old Age Psychiatry (Baldwin et al., 2003) is shown in Box 16.4.

When treatments seem to fail, some old age psychiatrists will suggest electroconvulsive therapy (ECT), a controversial treatment that involves triggering a convulsion by giving a powerful electric shock to the brain of the anaesthetised patient. There is an argument that ECT is more effective in older people than in younger people with depression, possibly at the price of worsening memory loss (Benbow, 2001).

Box 16.3   Recommendations for practice acute–treatment phase with antidepressants

- Older people with major depressive episode should be offered treatment with an antidepressant drug.
- For mild to moderate major depressive disorders, a psychological intervention can be offered as an effective alternative.
- For persistent minor depression (>4 weeks), a trial of antidepressant medication should be considered.
- Antidepressant treatment should be tailored to the individual, in terms of medication type and dosage.
- Older antidepressants (like the tricyclic group) should be avoided for people at risk of suicide.
- For people with major depression complicating dementia, treatment with an SSRI like Fluoxetine is recommended, along with increased support for the carer.
- For people with major illnesses as well as depression, the recommended antidepressants are SSRIs, Venlafixine, Mirtazepine, and Nefazodone.
- The use of low dosages of antidepressants in major depression is not recommended.
- With frail older people it is advisable to 'start low' and 'go slow' with antidepressant medication, using a low dose initially to ensure that the individual dose does not have any harmful adverse effects, and slowly increase it to the effective therapeutic dose.

Box 16.4 Treatment modality and type of depression

Type of depression	Treatment modality
Psychotic depression	Combined antidepressant or ECT–urgent referral indicated
Severe/major (non-psychotic) depression	Combined antidepressant and psychological therapy–consider referral
Mild–Moderate depressive episode	Antidepressant *or* psychological therapy (CBT, problem-solving, IPT or brief psychodynamic psychotherapy)
Dysthymia	Antidepressant
Recent-onset sub-threshold (minor) depression	Watchful waiting and support
Persistent sub-threshold (minor) depression	Antidepressant and support
Brief depression, grief reaction, and bereavement symptoms	Treat as for moderate depression if duration and intensity suggest intervention is indicated; otherwise support and watchful waiting
Persistent minor depression with comorbidity	Some evidence of the effectiveness of counselling

The use of Mental Health legislation for compulsory detention so that assessment and treatment can be carried out is not common among older people. Nurses, as other parts of this book explain, have particular roles and powers under mental health legislation, both inside in-patient units and in the community. Because older people are not often detained or subject to mental health legislation, not all nurses will have experience of these issues, and so learning from colleagues is important in ensuring that practice is legal, to advocate for older people, and to provide support to colleagues in the multidisciplinary team.

Information about older people's mental health is important to share, as Case Study 16.4 illustrates.

Case study 16.4

Mrs D has lived alone since her husband died 30 years ago, but she has friends who speak with her every day by phone, and visitors once or twice a week. She has been admitted to hospital with a hip fracture and seems fine after the operations, remobilizing after the surgery but is not remotivated. She has a history of depression. She is not sleeping well, often waking in the night and finding it difficult to return to sleep. She is asking for sleeping tablets. She looks depressed and admits to her nurse that life is not worth living. The nurse talks to the house officer, who raises the problem on the ward round. She is transferred to the rehab ward and advised to start antidepressants whilst remobilising. The care plan reflects these changes. The key nurse makes sure that in the ward transfer and discharge paperwork, the care team is alerted to the problems experienced by Mrs D and asks them to follow up the treatment of the depression.

While good practice seems now to be followed, this example raises the question of why Mrs D's history of depression was not known to the nursing staff. A previous history of depression increases the risk of it happening again, but recurrent depression in earlier life increases the likelihood that people will respond to antidepressants, although relapse is also likely. How did Mrs D cope when she was depressed before? The hospital staff have little available history, but they can alert their colleagues and, importantly, the primary care team to the need for follow-up of Mrs D.

Conclusion

Experienced nurses are able to think diagnostically and therapeutically about depression in later life. They can acknowledge the power and importance of an everyday approach to depression without idealising it, or understating its limitations. Depressed people (at any age) can be demanding and capable of triggering distress in those around them, who may avoid them because they are such hard work. Some people can deal easily with the emotional transference that can occur between the depressed individual and those in contact with them, but others may not be so capable. Nurses should be able to pass on their expertise, skills, and attitudes to care staff and carers, as well as being involved in treatment for older people with depression.

More education and training is often seen as the answer to everything, especially to problems that are hidden or under-recognised. Livingston et al. (2000) argue that training is not the main answer, and we suggest that capacity of services may be the area that should be developed further. Some of this can be inside health services, but commissioning of integrated services, and services in the voluntary and community sectors, may mean that older people with depression will be able to make use of services that are easily accessed and non-stigmatising. Local maps of services for older people with depression are worth compiling or commissioning, in part because there is no major campaigning group for older people with depression that undertakes such work.

It is often recognised that carers of depressed older people may be affected by the depressed mood that surrounds them. Sewitch et al. (2004) found that such carers need more psychosocial support because the depression of the person they are supporting may impact badly on their quality of life, and may worsen their own mental health. Carers may equally experience depression after they have ceased providing substantial support (Chene, 2006). The toll of depression on nurses and on teams needs also to be recognised. Nurses may discuss this in their work situation, and the mechanics of doing this should be clear, such as who will give mentoring and what workplace or occupational health support is available. The results of well-supported, paced and thoughtful clinical work with older people with depression can be dramatic, with abolition of debilitating physical symptoms, restoration of pleasure in everyday experience, and a step-change in their quality of life.

References

Alexopoulos, G.S., Katz, I.R., Reynolds, C.F., Carpenter, D. and Docherty, J.P. (2001) *The Expert Consensus Guideline Series: Pharmacotherapy of Depressive Disorders in Older Patients, Postgraduate Med Special Report (October), Expert Knowledge Systems, L.L.C.* Minneapolis, MN, McGraw-Hill Healthcare Information Programs, pp. 1–86.

Alzheimer's Society (2001) *Dementia in the Community: Management Strategies for Primary Care,* 2nd edn. London, Alzheimer's Society.

Audit Commission (2000) *Forget Me Not. London,* Audit Commission.

Bagley, H., Cordingley, L., Burns, A., Mozley, C., Sutcliffe, C., Challis, D. and Huxley, P. (2000) Recognition of depression by staff in nursing and residential homes. *Journal of Clinical Nursing* **9** (3), 445–450.

Baldwin, R., Anderson, D., Black, S., Evans, S., Jones, R., Wilson, K. and Iliffe, S. (2003) Guidelines for the management of late-life depression in primary care. *International Journal of Geriatric Psychiatry* **18** (9), 829–838.

Ballard C., Patel, A., Solis, M., Lowe, K. and Wilcock, G. (1996) A one-year follow-up study of depression in dementia sufferers. *British Journal of Psychiatry* **168**, 287–291.

Battison, T. (2004) *Caring for Someone with Depression.* London, Age Concern.

Beautrais, A. (2002) A case control study of suicide and attempted suicide among older adults. *Suicide and Life-Threatening Behaviour* **32** (1), 1–9.

Beekman, A., Copeland, J. and Prince, M. (1999) Review of community prevalence of depression in later life. *British Journal of Psychiatry* **174**, 307–311.

Beekman A., Kreigsman, D., Deeg, D. and Tilburg, W. (1995) The association of physical health and depressive symptoms in the older population: age and sex differences. *Social Psychiatry and Psychiatric Epidemiology* **30**, 32–38.

Benbow, S. (2001) ECT in the treatment of depression in older people. In: *Practical Management of Depression in Older People* (S. Curran, J. Wattis and S. Lynch, eds). London, Arnold, pp. 61–75.

Blanchard, M., Waterreus, A. and Mann, A. (2004) The effect of primary care nursing intervention upon older people screened as depressed. *International Journal of Geriatric Psychiatry* **10** (4), 289–298.

Boyle, V., Roychoudhury, C., Beniak, R., Cohn, L., Bayer, A. and Katz, I. (2004) Recognition and management of depression in skilled-nursing and long-term care settings *American Journal of Geriatric Psychiatry* **12**, 288–295.

Bracken, P., Greenslade, L., Griffin, B. and Smyth, M. (1998) Mental health and ethnicity: an Irish dimension. *British Journal of Psychiatry* **172**, 103–105.

Burns, A., Dening, T. and Baldwin, R. (2001) Care of older people: mental health problems. *British Medical Journal* **322**, 789–791.

Cattan, M. (2002) *Supporting Older People to Overcome Social Isolation and Loneliness.* London, Help the Aged.

Chene, B. (2006) Dementia and residential placement: a view from the carer's perspective. *Qualitative Social Work* **5** (2), 187–215.

Cheston, R. and Bender, M. (1999) *Understanding Dementia: The Man with the Worried Eyes.* London, Jessica Kingsley.

Chew-Graham, C., Baldwin, R. and Burns, A. (2004) Treating depression in later life. *British Medical Journal* **329**, 181–182.

de Leo, D., Padoani, W., Scocco, P., Lie, D., Bille-Brahe, U., Arensman, E., Hjelmeland, H., Crepet, P., Haring, C. and Hawton, K. (2001) Attempted and completed suicide in older subjects: results from the WHO/EURO multicentre study of suicidal behaviour. *International Journal of Geriatric Psychiatry* **16**, 300–310.

Department of Health (2001) *National Service Framework for Older People.* London, Department of Health.

Department of Health (2002) *National Suicide Prevention Strategy.* London, Department of Health.

Dyer, C., Pavlik, V., Murphy, K. and Hyman, D. (2000) The high prevalence of depression and dementia in elder abuse and neglect. *Journal of the American Geriatric Society* **48** (2), 205–208.

Eastman, M. (2005) In: *Moving out of the Shadows* (MOOTS) (H. Bowers, M. Eastman, J. Harris and A. Macadam, eds). Bournemouth, UK, Health and Care Development.

Fanthorpe, U.A. (1996) Walking in Darkness. In: *Mind Readings: Writers' Journeys through Mental States* (S. Dunn, B. Morrison and M. Roberts, eds). London, Minerva, pp. 51–54.

Garrard, J., Rolnick, S.J., Nitz, N.M. et al. (1998) Clinical detection of depression among community-based elderly people with self-reported symptoms of depression. *Gerontology* **53**, M92–M101.

Gottfries C.G. (2001) Late life depression. *European Archives of Psychiatry and Clinical Neuroscience* **251** (2), 73–79.

Harwood, D.M.J., Hawton, K., Hope, T. and Jacoby, R. (2000) Suicide in older people: mode of death, demographic factors, and medical contact before death. *International Journal of Geriatric Psychiatry*, **15**, 736–743.

Harwood, D.M.J., Hawton, K., Hope, T. and Jacoby, R. (2001) Psychiatric disorder and personality factors associated with suicide in older people: a descriptive and case control study. *International Journal of Geriatric Psychiatry* **16**, 155–165.

Highet, N., Thompson, M. and McNair, B. (n.d.) *The experiences and needs of carers and families living with depression.* http://www.arcvic.com.au/research/depressionfull

Katona, C.L.E. (1989) The epidemiology and natural history of depression in old age. In: *Antidepressants for Elderly People* (K. Ghose, ed.). London, Chapman & Hall.

Layard, R. (2004) *Mental health: Britain's biggest social problem?* http://www.strategy.gov.uk

Lebowitz, B., Pearson, J., Schnieder, L., Reynolds, C., Alexopoulos, G., Bruce, M., Conwell, Y., Katz, I., Myers, B., Morrison, M., Mossy, J., Niedereke, G. and Parmelee, P. (1997) Diagnosis and treatment of depression in late life: consensus statement update. *Journal of the American Medical Association* **278** (14), 1186–1190.

Levin E., Moriarty, J. and Gorbach, P. (1994) *Better for the Break.* London, HMSO.

Livingston, G., Yard, P., Beard, A. and Katona, C. (2000) A nurse-coordinated educational initiative addressing primary care professionals' attitudes to and problem-solving in depression in older people – a pilot study. *International Journal of Geriatric Psychiatry* **15** (5), 401–405.

Manthorpe, J. and Iliffe, S. (2005a) *Depression in Later Life.* London, Jessica Kingsley.

Manthorpe, J. and Iliffe, S. (2005b) Suicide and depression. *Nursing Older People* **17** (10), 25–29.

Manthorpe, J. and Iliffe, S. (2006) Depression and dementia: taking a dual diagnosis approach. *Nursing Older People* **18** (2), 24–29.

Marzanski, M. (2000) Would you like to know what is wrong with you? On telling the truth to patients with dementia. *Journal of Medical Ethics* **26**, 108–113.

Millard, P. (1983) Depression in old age. *British Medical Journal* **287**, 375–376.

Mills, T.L. and Edwards, C.D.A. (2002) A critical review of research on the mental health of older African-Americans. *Ageing and Society* **22**, 273–304.

Montano, C.B. (1999) Primary care issues related to the treatment of depression in elderly patients. *Journal of Clinical Psychiatry* **60**, 45–51.

Moriarty, J. and Webb, S. (2000) *Part of the Lives: Community Care for People with Dementia.* Bristol, UK, Policy Press.

Neal, M., Hughes, P. and Bell, M. (2001) The role of the nurse in the assessment, diagnosis and management of depression in older people. In: *Practical Management of Depression in Older People* (S. Curran, J. Wattis and S. Lynch, eds). London, Arnold, pp. 123–145.

O'Connell, H., Chin, A., Cunningham, C. and Lawlor, B. (2004) Recent developments: suicide in older people. *British Medical Journal* **329**, 895–899.

Office of the Deputy Prime Minister (2006) *Social Exclusion of Older People: Evidence from the First Wave of the English Longitudinal Study of Ageing (ELSA). New Horizons Research Summary No. 1, January.* London, The Stationery Office.

Owens, T., National Care Homes Research and Development Forum (2006) *My Home Life: Quality of Care in Care Homes.* London, Help the Aged.

Patmore, C. (2002) Morale and quality of life among frail older users of community care: key issues for the success of community care. *Quality in Ageing* **3**, 22–29.

Sewitch, M., McCustker, J., Dendukuri, N. and Yaffe, M. (2004) Depression in frail elders: impact on family caregivers. *International Journal of Geriatric Psychiatry* **19** (7), 655–665.

Sharma, V.K. and Copeland, J.R.M. (1989) Presentation and assessment of depression in old age. In: *Antidepressants for Elderly People* (K. Ghose, ed.). London, Chapman & Hall.

Turvey, C., Conwell, Y., Joes, M., Phillips, C., Simonsick, E., Rearson, J. and Wallace, R. (2002) Risk factors for late-life suicide: a prospective, community-based study. *American Journal of Geriatric Psychiatry* **10** (4), 398–406.

Waern, M., Rubenowitz, E., Runeson, B., Skoog, I., Wilheimson, K. and Allebeck, P. (2002) Burden of illness and suicide in elderly people: case control study. *British Medical Journal* **324**, 1355–1340.

Watts, S., Bhutani, G., Stout, I., Ducker, P., Cleator, P., McGarry, J. and Day, M. (2002) Mental health in older adult recipients of primary care services: is depression the key issue? Identification, treatment and the general practitioner. *International Journal of Geriatric Psychiatry* **17** (5), 427–437.

Wilkinson, P. (1997) Cognitive therapy with elderly people. *Age and Ageing* **26** (1), 53–58.

Chapter 17
Dementia in Later Life

Trevor Adams and Gary Blatch

Introduction

Nursing people with dementia is a practical activity and is best understood as something that nurses do. This approach displays a distrust of nurse academics who develop nursing theory that is far removed from the everyday work of nurses. Nevertheless, while nursing is primarily a practical activity, nurses should adopt a pragmatic and a critical and reflective approach that allows nurses to reflect upon what they are doing and generate new ways of working with people with dementia.

The approach adopted in this chapter draws on the ideas that developed in a school of sociology called 'ethnomethodology', which is concerned with how people make sense of and act in everyday practical situations within the social world (Dowling, 2006). Adopting this theoretical framework offers insights about how clinical situations in dementia care are understood and from which nurses make decisions.

Sometimes, people think of nursing people with dementia as a speciality. This understanding is problematic because it often makes nurses who do not generally work with people who have dementia feel as though they are outsiders and that they are ill-equipped and unskilled to work with people who have dementia. For nurses working outside specialist dementia care services, people with dementia are 'other people's business' and this is a great shame.

We would challenge this view and assert that dementia care is not just undertaken by one particular branch of nursing, say mental health nursing, but overlaps adult, mental health and learning disability nursing, and may occur in different settings such as in hospitals, the community, day hospitals and hospice settings. Nurses in all these settings repeatedly find themselves working with people who have dementia and from time to time will have responsibility for providing nursing care to people with dementia. The view that nurses working with people who have dementia are always registered mental health nurses leads to an inappropriate exclusivity within dementia care and impoverished care to people with dementia.

At the heart of dementia care nursing is the shared journey between the person with dementia, their family carer(s) and the dementia care nurse. At various parts of this journey, the nurse may know more about how the journey will progress and can help the person with dementia and/or their carer(s) deal with different things they find tricky. Every person with dementia and their family carer has the right to expect the best possible nursing care whether it is from a specialist dementia care unit or from an orthopaedic ward or Accident and Emergency Unit. This view of nursing people with dementia is affirmed by *Everybody's Business* (Department of Health and Care Services Improvement Partnership, 2005), which asserts that older people with mental health needs, including people with dementia, may be found in many sections of health care and that they should have the same expectation of good care as anyone else, including the right to dignity and optimal participation in decision-making. Nursing people with dementia is 'every nurse's business'.

Exploring dementia

Dementia is an acquired syndrome that is chronic, progressive and debilitating. The syndrome is characterised by global impairments that affect higher brain function. People with dementia find it difficult to do such things as remember what has happened to them, communicate with other people, and undertake different skilled social behaviour. Dementia is usually seen as a memory disorder comprising forgetfulness, primarily about recent events; orientation, regarding time, place and person; grasping items of new information; communication with other people; personality changes and behaviour disorders. However, it is more accurate to think of it as a wide range of physical, emotional, behavioural and social impairments that progressively undermine their ability to undertake socially accepted activities of everyday life.

The most common types of dementia are:

- Alzheimer's disease;
- vascular dementia;
- mild cognitive impairment;
- dementia with Lewy bodies;
- Binswanger's disease;
- frontotemporal dementia and Pick's disease.

Alzheimer's disease

Alzheimer's disease may take the form of either an early-onset familial disease (EOFAD) or a sporadic late-onset disease. Each of these forms of Alzheimer's disease is characterised by the occurrence of amyloid-containing extracellular plaques and the abnormal material that develops inside the neurones, the neurofibrillary tangles. It is thought that the degeneration of neurones may be caused by the deposition of amyloid beta-peptide in the brain tissue. EOFAD seems to be linked with three genes on chromosomes 21, chromosome 14q, and chromosome 1q. People with Alzheimer's disease have depleted levels of acetylcholine within transmitter fluids between neurones that recent pharmacological treatments such as donepezil and galantimine have sought to address. The clinical features of Alzheimer's disease are typical of those found in the dementia syndrome, though the condition usually has a slow onset.

Alzheimer's disease is characterised by:

- cognitive decline;
- gradual progression;
- intact level of consciousness;
- onset after the age of 40 years.

Alzheimer's disease is usually only recognised in retrospect and comprises impairment to memory (amnesia), coordination dexterity (apraxia), language (aphasia) and perception (agnosia). In the early stage of Alzheimer's disease, memory difficulties are predominant, and people may be troubled by forgetfulness and may develop personality changes. Later, people with Alzheimer's disease may find it difficult to use language, undertake everyday activities and recognise people, places and situations. During this stage, family carers may need to help the person go shopping and pay bills. In the later stages, people with Alzheimer's disease experience severe difficulty with their memory, praxis and recognising other people. They may also have difficulty walking and toileting, and gradually become dependent on other people for all their activities of daily living.

Vascular dementia

Vascular dementia gives rise to impaired cognition following a single stroke in a critical area of the brain such as the thalamus. Vascular dementia usually starts abruptly, recurrent small strokes may give rise to a typical stepwise progression and afterwards multiple infarcts may occur. Focal deficits may also occur and lead to neurological problems. It is not easy to distinguish between Alzheimer's disease and vascular dementia. While they are two different conditions, they often occur together, and when this happens they are described as 'a mixed dementia'. Only a post-mortem can confirm the diagnosis.

The development of dementia care nursing

As Chapter 1 describes, dementia care nursing has traditionally been underpinned by a 'warehousing' approach to care in which people with dementia are kept or housed for indefinite periods on long-stay wards in the hope that a cure may one day appear. This model viewed dementia as a disease and as having no environmental, psychological and social cause. Within this understanding of dementia, the aim of nursing people with dementia was institutional and concerned with maintaining the physical well-being of the person and maintaining order. In this coercive environment, there was little opportunity for people with dementia to control their own lives, and the provision of care was little more than physical care.

The marginalisation of people with dementia was, and still is, common in psychiatric nursing. As Professor Tony Butterworth notes 'working with elderly confused and dementing patients was, in my own training lifetime, used as a punishment for nurses who had overstepped the mark or committed an organisational misdemeanour' (Butterworth, 1998, p. 39). Marginalisation was endemic and was even fostered in nursing textbooks. For example, Houliston (1961, p. 122) states that 'a state of enfeeblement [was] due to disease or decay of the brain' and that '[U]nlike the mental defective who never was normal, the dement was normal once'.

Though institutionalisation still remains in some places, the move away from warehousing and institutional forms of dementia care began in the late 1960s. These developments were initiated by a small group of innovative psychiatrists who generated professional and academic interest in services for people with dementia and gave rise to innovative models of service delivery, most notably community mental health teams for older people. Whitehead (1970) describes such a team at Severalls Hospital, Essex, comprising different health care professionals working under a Consultant Psychiatrist. As a result of the growing interest in people with dementia within other health and social care professions, different approaches and insights have emerged and have been used to enhance the well-being of people with dementia.

At the same time, other changes were occurring, and an alternative and radical way of thinking about people with dementia was emerging. A key idea here was that people with dementia should be regarded as people rather than a diagnosis. This holistic approach emphasised that while people with dementia may have lost some cognition, ideas developed by Kitwood (1997) highlighted the need for staff such as nurses to undertake practices and activities that promote the personhood of people with dementia.

Of particular relevance to the recent development of services has been the National Service Framework (NSF) for Older People (Department of Health, 2001). This document is one of a number of frameworks that seek to enhance service provision by establishing various national standards. Standard 7 of the NSF for Older People deals with mental health, but while people with dementia were included in this standard, various agencies have argued that older people with dementia have received insufficient attention. This marginalisation of people with dementia was compounded by the failure of the NSF for Mental Health (Department of Health, 1999) to address the needs of people over the age of 65 years. As a result, people with dementia fell through the net and disappeared out of sight

Failing to highlight the needs of people with dementia was a clear mistake that may have contributed towards the continuation of poor standards. The poor standards of care on one ward, Rowan Ward, Withington Hospital Manchester, attracted the attention of the Commission for Health Improvement in October 2003. The Report, *Investigations Arising from Care on Rowan Ward Manchester Mental Health and Social Care Trust* (Commission for Health Improvement, 2003) outlined a list of bad practice that had occurred and identified various factors that had brought it about:

- geographical location;
- low staffing levels;
- lack of training;
- lack of nursing leadership;
- lack of clinical governance.

The publication of the report sent shock waves among health and social care professionals working with people who have dementia, and led the Department of Health to take urgent action to make sure that the same things would never happen again.

One action was to bridge the gap between mental health and dementia care that had been created within social policy. This was accomplished through the joint publication of *Securing Better Mental Health for Older Adults* (Department of Health, 2005) by the National Directors for Older People and Mental Health. In the publication, the two National Directors promoted the principles of:

- delivering non-discriminatory mental health and care services available on the basis of need, not age;
- holistic person-centred older people's health and care services that address mental as well as physical needs.

Everybody's business

Following the publication of *Securing Better Mental Health for Older Adults* (Department of Health, 2005), a second, more substantial document was published, *Everybody's Business* (Department of Health and Care Services Improvement Partnership, 2005). This latter document is a service development guide that lays out the main components of modern services for older people with mental health conditions.

The message put forward by Everybody's Business is best summarised in the key messages outlined for service commissioners below:

- older people's mental health is everybody's business;
- improving services for older people with mental health conditions will help meet national targets and standards;
- access to mental health services should not be based on age;
- older people need holistic care in mainstream services;
- workforce development is central to driving service improvement;
- whole-system commissioning and leadership are vital to deliver a comprehensive service.

While we would support many ideas contained in Everybody's Business, we cannot agree with all the ideas the Report contains, particularly those that advocate a 'generic' model of multi-disciplinary teamwork. This model argues that many of the skills needed to undertake dementia care are shared by different members of the multi-disciplinary team and fails to acknowledge the distinctive contributions made by different professionals. While we certainly do support multi-disciplinary teamwork, we believe that inter-professional and inter-agency collaboration is best displayed by recognising and valuing the distinctive contribution made by different health and social care professions to people with dementia and their families, not least nursing.

Governmental reviews of mental health nursing

In April 2006, the Chief Nursing Officer at the Department of Health published a review of the work of mental health nurses entitled From Values to Actions that sought to identify how the profession can best contribute to the care of service users in the future (Department of Health, 2006). At the same time, the Chief Nursing Officer of Scotland published a report *Rights, Relationships and Recovery* (Scottish Executive, 2006) that set out a similar, though different, statement about the nature of mental health nursing within contemporary society. Each of the two reviews was developed through consultation with users of a wide range of mental health services, family carers, nurses and representatives of various professional health- and social-care bodies, and makes key recommendations about mental health nursing.

While most of the recommendations are relevant to nurses working with people who have dementia, its support of the Recovery Approach sounds more applicable to the work of younger people with mental health conditions. Mental health nursing, adopts an inclusive approach that does not merely focus on people with dementia, and while the Recovery Approach may be an appropriate approach to use and is applicable to carers, it seems quite inappropriate with people with dementia.

However, while nursing people with dementia occurs in different types of clinical areas by a range of nurses, it is mental health nurses who are usually involved in specialist dementia services. For this reason, each of the reviews has considerable relevance for nursing people with dementia.

Dementia care nursing skills

But what are the skills that nurses need to work with people who have dementia and their families? These skills may be derived from a number of sources identifying the skills and competencies dementia care workers possess, as the works of Mace (2005), and Williams et al. (2005) highlight. These skills are discussed in the following subsections.

Cognitive skills

Two particular cognitive skills are used by nurses working with people who have dementia. The first is pattern recognition, through which nurses are able to view 'the bigger picture' in dementia care situations. This skill is gained by nurses repeatedly listening mand viewing situations and gaining a familiarity with them. The second skill is deduction and is the ability to elicit ideas and plans from a particular understanding of a practice situation (Case Study 17.1).

Case study 17.1

Joe was suspected of experiencing visual hallucinations because of his repeated descriptions of a man who 'went to the dining room with you' and 'had a really good sleep in that dormitory next to him' (pointing to Steve, a fellow resident). His visitors were concerned, but Joe seemed completely relaxed about it. He dismissed all questions about 'the man', clearly not understanding why we were asking questions and straining his relationships with others.

Having been in the dining room with Joe one lunchtime, I knew that Steve had been the only other person eating with Joe. I remembered that they had been talking animatedly, but I did not feel that Joe responded to the presence of another person next to him. I felt that Joe's 'other man' was possibly a symptom of word meaning being a problem for him. His descriptions seemed to have lost much of their accuracy because he had used a third-person perspective and completely changed their meaning. I spoke about this to the staff and his family, who could then develop a good understanding of the situation and no longer feel so distressed.

Dealing with uncertainty

There are many clinical situations, particularly in domiciliary care, that are unclear and ambiguous. Living with ambiguity may be difficult for some nurses, as there is a potential threat to their professional identity, if the client comes to any harm (Case Study 17.2).

Case study 17.2

Penny was recently married and was coming to terms with her new husband's recent diagnosis of Alzheimer's disease. She expressed fears that she would be 'unable to cope' if Steve, her husband, needed personal care or became 'unmanageable' I asked her whether she had discussed this with Steve, and Penny said that she 'could not', because she did not want to distress him- or herself.

I asked Penny and Steve what they thought their future held and arranged a return visit a couple days later. When I did so, it was clear that Penny had a very negative past experience observing her uncle, with dementia, some 40 years earlier. Steve had concerns that he knew 'almost nothing' about Alzheimer's disease and had no idea about the implications it had for him. I discussed in broad terms what was happening to Steve and tried to answer his questions constructively though honestly. I explained some of the options available to him and emphasised the opportunities that he had to share his wishes with others.

I discussed 'dementia drugs' at Penny's request and agreed to arrange an outpatient appointment for them both to discuss this with the consultant. I left the couple with literature from the Alzheimer's Society, to support what I had discussed, and arranged to return a few days later.

During further visits, I discussed the range of services and resources that were available to them locally and how they could access them. I gave Penny information about local carer-support groups, left them leaflets about benefits and allowances and discussed with Peter whether he would find it helpful to meet other people in his situation.

Communication

Nurses need to be able to talk easily with people. Barker et al. (1998) describes how knowledge elicited during assessments arises out of conversations that occur between people. Nurses working with people who have dementia and their family carer (s) need to use what they say and do, to generate information and accounts and stories that promote everybody's understanding about what is happening and contribute to decisions about options that are available (Case Study 17.3).

Case study 17.3

Russell had been described by staff as 'uncommunicative' and that he intimidated inexperienced staff by shouting seemingly inappropriately during attempted interactions. I spent some time with Russell and saw that his speech was sprinkled with sounds that did not resemble recognisable words. Staff spent much of their time working out what he was trying to say and would often not respond at all, wary of provoking him unintentionally.

I tried a combination of mirroring, and validation where I would repeat to him what I thought were his key words or points. Russell still took umbrage at my occasional misinterpretations of what he was attempting to say but, on the whole, communication with him improved and became more of a two-way process. It thus became much easier to know what he was saying and to address his wishes.

Diagnosis sharing and information giving

It is increasingly recognised that people with dementia have the same right to know their diagnosis as anyone else. Nurses may therefore find themselves in a position where they need to share the diagnosis of dementia and the implications it will have upon their life with a client and their relatives (Case Study 17.4).

Case study 17.4

Albert had recently been diagnosed as having vascular dementia. He lived alone, saw little of his family or friends and did not see any need to accept help from 'welfare'. He rarely wanted to talk about his memory difficulties, especially after outpatient appointments, but would sometimes ask me 'What is it that they think I have?' At the outpatient appointments, doctors had upset Albert by talking to him about 'dementia', so I tried to talk to him about having 'small strokes' rather than dementia. He seemed to understand the implications of this and was able to discuss the importance of taking his medication as well as realising why his memory often failed him. I hoped that by talking to him about this diagnosis and medication in a way he found acceptable that would foster Albert's trust and allow further work helping him come to terms with his condition and helping him make realistic plans for the future.

Physical nursing skills

Recent developments in dementia have tended to focus on the psychological nature of dementia. However, nurses need to acknowledge that people with dementia are embodied and have bodily needs that arise partly from dementia and partly through normal ageing and different pathological processes. Nurses therefore need skills associated with providing physical care (Case Study 17.5).

Case study 17.5

Delia lived with her husband, who was also her primary carer, assisting her with most of her personal care. He told me that she normally enjoyed his meals but now, at tea times, she needed help to eat and did not seem so keen, often rejecting his attempts to offer her food. I watched one mealtime and noticed that he stood behind her silently, bending down to offer her the fork. Delia was making very negative sounds and pulling her head away from the fork. I suggested that he should sit down at the table next to her, putting himself at her left-hand side and at her level. I also suggested he talked to her in the same way as he did when they ate together previously. Delia appeared to be more at ease when these suggestions were put into practice. As an observer, I felt she regained her dignity, and felt less of a passive participant and that mealtimes returned to being a social occasion again.

Integrating different perspectives

There is more than just one way of seeing what is happening or what should happen. Nurses should try to help the person with dementia and their family carer(s) come to a shared and agreed decision so that both parties feel that they have gained something and that they are contributing to the situation moving forward (Case Study 17.6).

Case study 17.6

Louisa lived alone and was fiercely independent. She wanted to remain in the house she had bought with her late husband 50 years before. She was adamant that she would 'die in that house before they drag me out of it'. She cooked for herself, kept her house clean, albeit untidy and visited the local shops every day for her food.

Louisa's daughter, Tracey, lived an hour away and had concerns that her mother was 'going to die if she's left to her own devices', saying how Louisa had left her key behind many times when she went out shopping, no longer paid bills and 'wears the same filthy clothes all week'. Louisa's GP saw the situation the same way. He felt the situation was unsafe, saw the unchanged clothes as a sign of self-neglect and referred Louisa to the local community mental health team. As the Community Mental Health Nurse, I was asked to visit to assess the situation and support Louisa and Tracey.

From a person-centred standpoint, I wanted to intervene only as much as was necessary to ensure that Louisa was safe. A key safe fitted to the door – and the combination given to her kind and long-term friend – meant that she would be less likely to lock herself out. I suggested that Tracey should discuss with her mother the possibility of taking out an enduring power of attorney, having utility bills redirected to her house and therefore being able to ensure all bills are paid and feel as though she was being of practical help to her mother. Louisa was happy to agree to this, on the understanding that she still had enough money to do her own shopping.

I suggested that her reluctance to change clothes was not something that bothered Louisa too much and probably reflected a change in priorities for her, rather than being self-neglect. My aim in future visits would be to encourage Tracey to support her mother's abilities and helping her accept that fulfilling her mother's wishes involves a certain degree of risk.

Networking and developing a shared approach to care

Different people and agencies contribute to promoting the well-being of the person with dementia and their family carer(s). This means that effective communication and networking should exist between people with dementia, their family carer(s) and different health and social care workers from statutory, voluntary, private and informal agencies. Nurses have an important role in fostering good networking and communication (Case Study 17.7).

Case study 17.7

Rachel lived with her retired and widowed daughter, Anna, in a small bungalow. Rachel had dementia, and Anna spent a great deal of time and love striving to keep a healthy relationship between them despite Rachel's severe difficulty in expressing herself.

Anna found that her mother often settled very quickly when agitated if she 'found' a realistic doll that had been Anna's when very young. I had discussed this with Anna, who felt that it gave her mother pleasure, seemed to foster a sense of caring and encouraged conversation. It became a sticking point during respite care when staff would discourage Anna from bringing in the doll or, worse, prevent other staff from giving it to her, as they felt it was 'patronising and undignified'.

I decided to raise this issue at the forthcoming review of Rachel's care package. I spoke briefly on 'doll therapy' and shared a case study I had read from a nursing journal. The manager of the home felt sure that her staff would now see the doll in a different light and invited Anna and I to her next staff meeting. Rachel's social worker included the doll in Rachel's care plan and said she would ensure that any forthcoming sitting services would also be made aware. A shared approach is generally easier to achieve when stakeholders meet together.

Case management

An important skill that nurses need when working with people who have dementia and their family carers is the ability to organise their work. In hospital and residential settings, some of the tasks relating to case management may be undertaken by senior staff working with people who have dementia, though some tasks such as record keeping and the management of individual clients may need to be appropriately managed. In the community settings, case management is often more complex (Case Study 17.8).

Case study 17.8

Jason lived on his own and was maintained by a social network that ensured his safety, needs and some of his wants. Jason had frontal-lobe dementia, which often resulted in him being 'unpredictable' and vulnerable. He was very wary of 'strangers' and rarely remembered even his close friends if he had not seen them for a while. He often rang the 'wrong' people to ask a question or enquire about an appointment, giving up when he heard someone say: 'You need to ring this person instead … .'

Some way of linking individuals and agencies so that they would not overlap or omit services but also informed each other of their existence was needed.

Case study 17.8   (Continued)

As such the Care Programme Approach (CPA) was adopted.

However, Jason was concerned that the service agencies would 'mess about with it all' during the CPA meeting, but we explained to him why we were there, that he would notice nothing changing from day to day, and that he would now only have one number to ring. I would make sure the recipient received his message. The care co-ordinator approach takes more time but, especially when mental health needs are complex, helps ensure a seamless service with efficient communication.

Conclusion

This chapter has been concerned with the future direction of dementia care nursing and has linked recent important social policy such as that contained in Everybody's Business (Department of Health and Care Services Improvement Partnership 2005) and the Reviews of Mental Health Nursing with discussion about the skills base required to do this work. However, we do not believe the discussion should end here but rather that a great amount of work is still to be done to address substantial workforce issues that exist in dementia care nursing such as the need to increase the attractiveness of working with people who have dementia and the need to set up education and training programmes that will help dementia care nurses enhance the skill they have available to work with people who have dementia such as their ability to communicate effectively with them as a means of enhancing their physical and emotional well-being (Adams, 2006; Surr, 2006). Addressing these needs should be set within the wider socio-political context, and it should be recognised that there needs to be a much greater provision of direct resources by government agencies such as the National Institute of Mental Health and Care Services Improvement Partnership to developing the workforce within dementia care and thus enhancing the quality of care.

References

Adams, T. (2006) *The Report of the Second Stage of the Oldercare Practice Development Project*. Guildford, UK, University of Surrey.

Barker, P.J., Reynolds, B. and Stevenson, C. (1998) The human science basis of psychiatric nursing: theory and practice. *Journal of Advanced Nursing* **25**, 660–667.

Butterworth, T. (1998) Breaking the boundaries. *Nursing Times* **34**, 36–39.

Commission for Health Improvement (2003) *Investigation into Matters Arising from Care on Rowan Ward*. London, Manchester Mental Health and Social Care Trust.

Department of Health (1999) *National Service Framework for Mental Health*. London, The Stationery Office.

Department of Health (2001) *National Service Framework for Older People*. London, The Stationery Office.

Department of Health and Care Services Improvement Partnership (2005) *Everybody's Business*. London, The Stationery Office.

Department of Health (2005) *Securing Better Mental Health for Older Adults.* London, The Stationery Office.

Department of Health (2006) *From Values to Actions, Review of Mental Health Nursing.* London, The Stationery Office.

Dowling, M. (2006) Ethnomethodology: Time for a revisit? A discussion paper. International Journal of Nursing Studies (in press).

Houliston, M. (1961) *The Practice of Mental Nursing.* Edinburgh, E & S Livingstone.

Kitwood, T. (1997) *Dementia Reconsidered. Buckingham,* UK, Open University Press.

Mace, N. (2005) *Teaching Dementia Care: Skill and Understanding.* Baltimore, MD, Johns Hopkins University Press.

Scottish Executive (2006) *Rights, Relationships and Recovery.* London, The Stationery Office.

Surr, C.A. (2006) Preservation of self in people with dementia living in residential care: a social-biographical approach. *Social Science and Medicine* **62**, 1720–1730.

Whitehead, A. (1970) *In Service of Older Age.* Harmondsworth, UK, Pelican.

Williams, C.L., Hyer, K., Kelly, S., Leger-Krall, S. and Tappen, R.M. (2005) Developments of nurse competencies to improve dementia care. *Geriatric Nursing* **26** (2), 98–105.

Part 5
FUTURE DIRECTIONS

Chapter 18
Mental Health and Well-Being for Older People in the Future: The Nursing Contribution

Henry Minardi, Hazel Heath and Rebecca Neno

Introduction

Predicting the future for older people's mental health and well-being is difficult. While we broadly know how many people are likely to enter older age in the foreseeable future, we cannot predict what health issues these people might encounter or how they will experience these.

Predicting future agendas for mental health services is even more difficult. This becomes apparent when we consider the rapidity of change within our localities, but more so as we acknowledge how national and international political and social agendas are changing. What happens in the world has an impact on national and local issues, particularly in terms of the migration of people who could become our clients or work colleagues.

This chapter discusses demographic trends and what might influence the mental health and well-being of future generations of older people. It considers emerging issues concerning the mental health of older people, including some not yet widely recognised. How policies and services are developing around the UK is acknowledged, and the chapter concludes by signposting key contributions that nursing could make to older people's mental health and well-being in the future.

Future populations of older people and nurses

As mental health conditions are not an inevitable aspect of ageing, there is no reason to suppose that the majority of older people in the future will not continue to enjoy good mental health and make valuable contributions to society, as they do now. If the current prevalence of mental health needs remains, the numbers of older people experiencing mental health conditions will increase proportionately as the numbers of older people in the UK increase. Age Concern and the Mental Health Foundation (2006) highlight this in predicting that, by 2021, over three million pensioners will experience mental health problems unless action is taken to promote good mental health and well-being for older people.

As societies evolve, and new populations come into later life, concepts of mental health could change. Age Concern England and the Mental Health Foundation (2004) suggest that mental health is not only an individual construct but also embedded within social relations and the construction of the societies within which we live, with all of the factors that enhance or undermine it. The characteristics, needs and aspirations of future generations of older people will be different from those who are old now. These people could be more vocal and politically aware, more widely travelled, more active and have a higher need for stimulation (Ask the Experts, 2006). This will require rethinking in order to plan services appropriate and acceptable to this group.

Information technology (IT) is an increasingly significant influence as its potentials become ever more diverse and its use becomes more widespread. Millions of people currently use the Internet for a variety of reasons (New Scientist, 2006). Older people, it is suggested, use it mainly to gather information, while younger people also use it for social networking (Gefter, 2006). The consequences of this for the future are that not only will older adults, on average, be more knowledgeable about their health than the present cohorts of older adults, but changes in planning activities, socialising or shopping are more likely to occur as a result of increased Internet usage.

Another major trend is the increasing diversity of the older population, for example in terms of ethnicity. Age Concern (2006) estimate that by 2030, the minority ethnic elder population in the UK will have increased tenfold, from 175 000 to over 1.7 million. The greatest part of that increase will take place in the next 15 years. The cultural diversity in some areas is particularly rich, and London currently has the highest proportion of people from minority ethnic groups (Age Concern, 2006), but there has also been significant migration to small towns in Britain, such as Leominster, Slough and Peterborough from new members of the European Union (Swinford, 2006). Although Swinford's article focuses on young, fit migrants, there are two predictable developments from this; first that these individuals will age, eventually becoming part of the group now labelled 'elderly' and second that a proportion will develop some form of mental health need, as can be expected in the general population at present.

Significant numbers of nurses within the UK workforce are from overseas and although the number has dropped in the past two years, many still want to come to the UK. Currently, approximately one in 12 nurses across the UK and one in four in Greater London come from overseas and again, the cultural mix in some areas is particularly rich. In one study for the Royal College of Nursing (Buchan, 2003), one London NHS Trust reported employing nurses from 68 nationalities.

Because, in the reality of Britain's health and social care, most service users are older, the majority of nurses coming from overseas will be working with older people, even if this is not their first choice. The importance of developing multi-cultural awareness, understanding and sensitivity cannot be overstated.

For example, with older people whose language or cognitive functioning is impaired, non-verbal communication, such as body language, exhibited by those who care for them can be misinterpreted resulting in negative perceptions of care received. Also, nurses who come from countries where communal care homes for older people do not exist may experience particular challenges in trying to work within such environments.

The mental health and well-being of older people in the future

Along with the proportional increase in mental health needs among older age groups, there will also likely be an increase in the number of 'graduates'. These would be people already in the mental health system with conditions such as severe and enduring mental illness, manic depression and obsessive-compulsive disorder, who have now reached pensionable age, and their mental health needs would be better met by an older adult mental health team. However, an increase in the prevalence of newly identified mental health needs may also emerge, including those often not identified as issues among older adults.

Alcohol dependence in older adults at present has an overall prevalence of up to 5% in community populations, rising to 12% in men aged 60 (Dyson, 2006). However, it is under-reported as an issue with older adults (Older People's Programme, 2006) often because health care workers do not think of 'ordinary' older adults as having an alcohol problem, only 'down and outs'. The numerous stresses some older adults are often placed under, for example, multiple bereavements, physical illness, financial loss or reduced income, ageist attitudes or loneliness and isolation, are sometimes viewed as appropriate reasons for having 'a drink or two', without thinking there may be a problem. Again, with an increase and changes in presentation of the older population, a change in the way mental health nurses view and care for older adults who drink in excess will need to be developed.

More people who have used or are still using illegal substances are likely to enter the health care system at some point. Thus problems such as cannabis-induced psychosis (Hides et al., 2006) which are common in older people may start to be experienced by people over the age of 65 and therefore contact with mental health nurses should be expected. Caring for older adults with drug-related issues will challenge the resourcefulness of younger nurses who assume that such issues could not relate to older adults. Thus, new ways of working with older people who present with these issues will require nurses to adapt and change from the way they currently work with older adults.

Other groups identified for 'special 'consideration by the Department of Health (2006a) were:

- younger people with dementia;
- older people with learning disabilities;
- mental health care for older prisoners.

The Alzheimer's Society (2005) estimates that in the UK, there are over 18 000 people under the age of 65 with some type of dementia including vascular dementia, fronto-temporal dementia, dementia with Lewy bodies, alcohol-related brain impairment or Korsakoff's syndrome and rarer forms such as Creutzfeldt–Jakob Disease. People with other conditions such as Parkinson's disease, Huntington's disease or multiple sclerosis may also develop dementia as part of their illness. Although symptoms of dementia may be similar, whatever a person's age, younger people often have different needs and encounter significant age-related barriers trying to access dementia services.

People with learning disabilities are living longer than ever before, and for approximately 50%, life expectancy is on a par with the general population. In later life, they consequently experience the effects of the ageing process, including multiple pathologies, alongside their learning disability. People with Down's syndrome show premature ageing and are particularly susceptible to Alzheimer's disease and a range of long-term health conditions. Older people with learning disabilities need the same kind of support as younger people but often receive less help. Staff with experience of working with older people often have not received training in learning disability. Similarly, staff working with older people with learning disabilities have training needs relating to the effects of ageing (Foundation for People with Learning Disabilities, 1999).

In a study for the Prison Reform Trust, Howse (2003) estimated that more than half of older people suffer from a mental health condition, the most common being depression as a result of imprisonment. Overall, their health is worse than that of their peers in the community. Many have no family or community links, and regime concessions such as less strenuous exercise classes are granted in less than a quarter of prisons. The majority of prisons do not have facilities to cope with people who have mobility problems or with impairments. Between 1990 and 2000, the number of sentenced older prisoners trebled, and both the number and proportion of older prisoners serving long sentences have increased significantly. These increases are not explained by demographic changes or any so-called 'elderly crime wave', but by harsher sentencing policies. Howse (2003) suggests that the courts are tending to imprison those older offenders whose crimes most challenge society's age-related stereotypes. It is now being recognised that older prisoners are not receiving the appropriate health care they need (Carlisle, 2006). Discussions in the House of Commons and reports by Podmore (2006a, b) warn that our failure to tackle widespread mental ill health among prisoners will contribute to social and public health issues for the future.

Other emerging mental health priorities among older people have been identified by the UK Inquiry into Mental Health and Well-being in Later Life conducted by the Older People's Programme (2006) as:

- people with both mental health and physical health problems;
- carers of people with dementia;
- older women, especially those experiencing abuse or domestic violence;

- homeless older people (discussed in Chapter 15);
- older people living in a care home (also identified as a priority by Age Concern and Mental Health Foundation, 2006).

Developments in treatment and care

The future approaches to prevention, treatment and care for older people with mental health issues will be profoundly influenced by developments in drugs, therapeutic measures, equipment and technology. The value and uses for Assistive Technology (AT) are likely to become better understood, as its use becomes more widespread, as with developments such as Telecare (Rice, 2005). Telecare involves technology which enables the monitoring of individuals by care professionals from a distance, detecting, for example, motion, falls, fire or gas and triggering a warning to a response centre. It is, however, also important not to rely solely on telecare, as the social contact and the maintenance of social networks are thought to contribute to health and well-being and can facilitate early recognition of behaviour changes such as those caused by depression or dementia. Also, although recognising that there are advantages in using technology, there are possible dangers such as a potential for fraudulent practices when the Internet is used by vulnerable older adults. None the less, from their 2004 review, Age Concern and the Mental Health Foundation concluded that there is limited but positive evidence that use of new technologies such as the Internet and videophones can promote mental health in later life.

Key underpinning principles of the development of assistive technologies seem to include creating and sustaining social networks, learning new skills and maintaining contact with family members, many of whom may be dispersed geographically. The roles for mental health nurses will be vast but may include encouraging older adults to use available technology where appropriate, monitoring of health via assistive technology and coaching and supporting older people in its usage.

Developing services for the future

The changing characteristics of people coming into older age identified above must prompt re-examination of the services offered in the future and the settings within which care should be available to older adults with mental health issues. For example, at the moment it is frequently suggested that some clients with very disruptive behaviour cannot or should not be cared for in present services for older adults (defined as over 65 years old). However, can this remain a viable option if the numbers increase as the demographic shift implies? Even though it is has been found in some populations of older adults that symptom presentation is dampened by age (Keogh and Roche, 1996), this cannot be assumed to be the case for those individuals who reach later life in the future.

Everybody's Business: Integrating Mental Health Services for Older Adults: A Development Guide, the Department of Health (2006a) identified a range of services for older adults with mental health issues that require development. These include:

- primary and community care: (primary care, home care, day services, housing,
- assistive technology and telecare and care in residential settings);
- intermediate care;
- care for people in the general hospital;
- other specialist mental health services (integrated community mental health teams, memory assessment services, psychological therapies and in-patient care).

New initiatives also offer opportunities. For example, 'Payment by results' is a new form of funding within the NHS in England that has been summarised by Carpenter (2006, p. 1): 'Reimbursement of hospital activity will be based on counting the number of patients, appropriately coded into groups whose treatments should cost the same, wherever they are treated.' This should see an end to the postcode lottery of health care within the UK, but the potential effect of this on older adults with mental health issues is likely to be indirect rather than direct. For example, although it is recommended by the Chief Nursing Officer Review of Mental Health (Department of Health, 2006b) that nurses caring for older people with mental health needs access further training in specific forms of intervention such as Cognitive-Behavioral Therapy, they are less likely to be seconded to do this as other professionals are already in place, such as clinical psychologists, to undertake this work. However, if new interventions can demonstrate cost-effectiveness, they are more likely to be funded. An example would be Home Treatment Teams (McNab et al., 2006), which provide a community-based service for older adults, something the present government supports.

Other initiatives are also being developed throughout the UK. The Mental Health and Well-being in Later Life Programme works in collaboration with the Scottish Executive (2003a) and other agencies to improve the health and well-being of older people across Scotland by developing a comprehensive programme of work to highlight good practice, raise awareness of the issues and support innovative initiatives. It encompasses workshops, education for participation courses, research and dissemination (for example into older people's perceptions of mental health and well-being in later life), regional interest groups and building capacity through local schemes. The programme also worked with the Centre for Research on Families and Relationships on an investigation and report on Older Women and Domestic Violence in Scotland, published in May 2003 (Scottish Executive, 2003b). In Wales, the *Strategy for Older People* (Welsh Assembly Government, 2003), a National Service Framework (NSF), focusing on health and social care services for older people, has now been developed.

Although there is currently no equivalent to the NSF for older people in Northern Ireland (NI), similar issues are being addressed through different strategies. A review of the Mental Health Order for NI is taking place and standards to improve services for mental health, including dementia and learning disabilities are currently being developed by the Social Services Inspectorate.

Nursing in the future

Priorities for nursing older adults who have mental health needs have been identified by the Chief Nursing Officer for England (Department of Health, 2006b).

Developing approaches that genuinely form partnerships in care with clients and their carers

The UK Inquiry into Mental Health and Well-being in Later Life conducted by the Older People's Programme (2006) sought information about the lived experience of older people with mental health difficulties and others with a range of mental health experiences and expectations, including carers. It highlights what works and what does not work, as well as some of the important similarities and differences around the UK. Their overwhelming finding was that the voices of older people and of carers about mental health experiences and aspirations are at best very quiet and at worst non-existent. There is a very low level of awareness of, and understanding about, older people's experiences, knowledge, confidence and understanding in the literature and practice developments. These findings impact upon the ability to work in partnership with clients and their carers. To achieve such therapeutic partnerships, strong relationships need to be developed with both clients and their carers so that a true understanding of their needs can be formulated.

There is a vast literature on support for carers, and Age Concern and the Mental Health Foundation (2004) conclude that the greatest effects of the development of therapeutic partnerships and intervention seem to be an increase in carers' knowledge, improved respite provision and consequent increases in social networks. There is often an immense sense of loss associated with caring in later life, and initiatives that focus on dealing with loss could prove effective in improving the mental health and well-being of carers.

Recognising and acting on the lack of service choices or even provision for users who are old

This becomes even more difficult if there is a physical health issue such as deafness or visual impairment that requires attention as well as a mental health need. Mental health nurses need to be able to recognise and care for the physical health needs of their clients, but also know limitations and when referral is appropriate. Mental health nurses also need to be able to provide appropriate and effective psychological therapies or interventions which are theoretically informed.

Facilitating social inclusion, social support and meeting spiritual needs

Nurses need to seek ways of helping older people to remain engaged within their communities and recognise the importance of meeting spiritual needs. Age Concern and the Mental Health Foundation (2004) conclude that all the evidence points to the positive influence of spirituality and religious belief on mental health in later life, as well as the importance of individual and social support, sense of purpose and being able to let go of one's worries and responsibilities. There is a sense that coming to terms with mortality is aided by a spiritual context. A belief system is not an intervention, and for those who do not subscribe, it cannot be imposed. Nevertheless, the benefits conferred by membership, however loosely defined, in a community of faith, are consistent with what we know about the promotion of mental health.

Developing the evidence base for practice

There will be more emphasis on basing practice on evidence, so mental health nurses will need to consider interventions in relation to papers which research and evaluate these interventions. This is not meant to stifle creativity but to consider how a new or different intervention can be evaluated, thus allowing its use to be defended. This will require nurses in the future to be genuinely widely read and not just rely on participation in formal education and training events. More nurses need to understand and undertake research to widen the pool of available research-based evidence. Of equal importance is the interpretation, analysis and synthesis of research findings and the implementation of these into practice, if appropriate, for the benefit of clients.

Nurses caring for older adults with mental health needs will have to become more self-reflective and analyse the practices of colleagues from their own and other disciplines with whom they work. In conjunction with this practice, they will need to be productively assertive with nursing and other colleagues in the best interests of clients. This will require the development of effective leadership, management and coaching skills in the future, and is a new challenge that both health and education must embrace.

Addressing challenges in professional practice

These developments will require the construction of a new skill set often not associated with nursing. Nurses will need to become business-orientated, they will need to demonstrate that they understand the cost of health and social care and be able to demonstrate its worth for clients. With the introduction of commissioning within England (Department of Health, 2005), nurses may find themselves in unfamiliar territory. As Primary Care Trusts split into provider and commissioning arms, there is no requirement for Primary Care Trusts to commission current provider services. This has created exciting and unprecedented opportunities for nurses, who may develop entrepreneurial practices and social enterprises. These developments have created tension within the nursing profession, as some question whether nurses can balance the requirements of business against the delivery of high-quality person-centred care. Nonetheless, it appears that this policy direction is here to stay, for the time being at least, and nurses must seize the opportunities to safeguard effective and evidence-based care for older adults with mental health needs.

To achieve this will require the development of skills such as influencing and negotiating, which can be utilised across a number of situations within both the client and multiprofessional context. It is paramount that nurses develop a 'voice' so that they can articulate best practice and make cases for expenditure and care within a business-driven NHS to ensure all older adults with mental health needs receive appropriate and timely care and treatment.

Challenges relating to clinical practices are also set to continue, as role boundaries continue to blur, and roles continue to expand. In recent years, nurses caring for older adults with mental health needs have seen an unprecedented increase in their skills and abilities, including the introduction of independent prescribing and treatments.

Conclusion

The importance of mental health and well-being will increase in the future as older people become statistically more significant in the population. It will be important for mental health nurses to recognise that this future older population will have different characteristics from the present population. It will be vital to recognise increasing diversity when engaging with individuals and communities, education being fundamental in supporting this.

The evidence suggests that interventions are still driven by the perceptions of policy-makers and researchers (Age Concern and the Mental Health Foundation, 2004). Most conspicuous in the literature is the sense that people in later life themselves have not had any input into the design or delivery of interventions for the promotion of their own mental health. What positive mental health means to individuals must be examined (Older People's Programme, 2006). Above all, we need to 'amplify and really listen to the diverse voices of older people with different mental health needs, experiences, aspirations and expectations'. It is important to acknowledge that mental health needs exist across the life course. This includes addressing social inequities, social isolation and mental health promotion recognising the need for meaningful social engagement with communities and that there is a close association between deprivation, poverty and mental health.

The Older People's Programme (2006, p. 9) states:

'A radical and wide-sweeping reform is needed to engage with and respond to the expressed needs and aspirations of older people and carers about mental health and the kinds of support that make a positive difference to well-being. Only by acting together – across political, cultural, sectors, communities and service agendas can we hope to shift attitudes and mindsets about mental health and well-being in later life.'

As Crump (1998, p 170) observes:

'to stand still, in other words to stop thinking and developing, in any climate is to start sliding backwards. If individuals begin to think they have achieved the best service for older people with mental health needs the care they offer has already begun to move backwards. If thought is part of the forward movement of care, absence of thought creates stagnation and ultimate backward movement in care.'

Nurses clearly have a central and crucial role to play.

References

Age Concern (2006) *Black and minority ethnic elders: fact and figures.* http://www.ageconcern.org.uk

Age Concern England and the Mental Health Foundation (2004) *Literature and policy review for the joint inquiry into mental health and well-being in later life.* http://www.mphilli.org/documents/litandpolicyreviewexecsummary.pdf

Age Concern England and the Mental Health Foundation (2006) *Promoting Mental Health and Well-Being in Later Life. A First Report from the UK Inquiry into Mental Health and Well-Being in Later Life.* London, Age Concern England and the Mental Health Foundation.

Alzheimer's Society (2005) *Younger People with Dementia: Information Sheet.* London, Alzheimer's Society.

Ask the Experts (2006) Future perfect or imperfect? *Nursing Older People* **18** (9), 23–24.

Buchan, J. (2003) Here to stay? *International Nurses in the UK.* London, Royal College of Nursing.

Carlisle, D. (2006) So far, so bleak. *Nursing Older People* **18** (7), 21–23.

Carpenter, I. (2006) Payment by results, in a nutshell. *British Geriatric Society Newsletter*, Issue 7, September, 1–3.

Crump, A. (1998) Disease or distress. In: *Caring for Older People: Developing Specialist Practice* (J. Marr and B. Kershaw, eds). London, Arnold, pp. 165–189.

Department of Health (2005) *Commissioning a Patient Led NHS.* London, Department of Health.

Department of Health (2006a) *Everybody's Business. Integrated Mental Health Services for Older Adults: a Service Development Guide.* London, Department of Health.

Department of Health (2006b) *From Values to Action: The Chief Nursing Officer's Review of Mental Health Nursing.* London, Department of Health.

Dyson, J. (2006) Alcohol misuse and older people. *Nursing Older People* **18** (7), 32–35.

Foundation for People with Learning Disabilities (1999) *Older People with Learning Disabilities: Review of the Literature.* Updates, vol. 1, issue 4. London, Foundation for People with Learning Disabilities.

Gefter, A. (2006) This is your space. *New Scientist* **191**, 25659, 46–48.

Hides, L., Dawe, S., Kavanagh, D.J. and Young, R.M. (2006) Psychotic symptoms and cannabis relapse in recent-onset psychosis: Prospective study. *The British Journal of Psychiatry* **189** (2), 137–143.

Howse, K. (2003) *Growing old in prison.* http://www.prisonreformtrust.org.uk

Keogh, F. and Roche, A. (1996) *Mental Disorders in Older Irish People: Incidence, Prevelance and Treatment, Report No. 45.* Dublin, National Council for the Elderly.

McNab, L., Smith, B. and Minardi, H. (2006). A new service in the intermediate care of older adults with mental health problems. *Nursing Older People* **18** (3), 22–26.

Older People's Programme (2006) *Disregarded and Overlooked: Report from the 'Learning from Experience' Research into the Needs, Experiences, Aspirations and Voices of Older People with Mental Health Needs and Carers across the UK.* London, Older People's Programme.

Podmore, J. (2006a) Trapped inside. *The Guardian*, 15 November 2006. Society@Guardian. co.uk

Podmore, J. (2006b) *Prison mental health care must be a major priority for the NHS. SCMH lecture*, 15 November 2006. http://www.scmh.org.uk

Rice, T. (2005) New solutions for ageing problems. *Nursing Older People* **17** (1), 10–12.

Scottish Executive (2003a) *National Programme for Improving Mental Health and Well-Being: Action Plan 2003–2006.* Edinburgh, Scottish Executive.

Scottish Executive (2003b) *Investigation and report on older women and domestic violence in Scotland.* http://www.healthscotland.com/topics/stages/healthy-ageing/mental-health-later-life.aspx#research

Swinford, S. (2006) How many others can we squeeze in? *The Sunday Times*, http://www.timesonline.co.uk/tol/news/uk/article62073.ece 27 August.

Welsh Assembly Government (2003) *Strategy for Older People in Wales.* Cardiff, Welsh Assembly Government.

Index

Note: Page numbers in *italics* represent figures, those in **bold** represent tables.